Industry and HMOs:
A Natural Alliance

INDUSTRY AND HEALTH CARE 5

Industry and HMOs:
A Natural Alliance

Edited by
Richard H. Egdahl and
Diana Chapman Walsh

Springer-Verlag New York

Springer Series on Industry and Health Care
Richard H. Egdahl, M.D., PhD.
Diana Chapman Walsh, M.S.
Center for Industry and Health Care
Boston University Health Policy Institute
53 Bay State Road
Boston, Massachusetts 02215

Springer-Verlag New York Inc.
175 Fifth Avenue
New York, New York 10010

Library of Congress Cataloging in Publication Data
Main entry under title:

Industry and HMOs—a natural alliance.

(Springer series on industry and health care; no. 5)
1. Health maintenance organizations—United States. 2. Labor and laboring classes—Medical care—United States. 3. Health maintenance organizations—United States—Congresses. 4. Labor and laboring classes—Medical care—United States—Congresses. I. Walsh, Diana Chapman. II. Egdahl, Richard Harrison.
RA413.5.U5I5   362.1'04'25   78-10912

© 1978 by Springer-Verlag New York Inc.

Printed in the United States of America

9 8 7 6 5 4 3 2 1

ISBN 0-387-90366-6 Springer-Verlag New York Heidelberg Berlin
ISBN 3-540-90366-6 Springer-Verlag Berlin Heidelberg New York

Preface

This fifth issue in the Industry and Health Care series takes a quick turn through unpredictable and only partially charted waters. The series as a whole has set out to explore the role of industry as a potential agent of change in the health care system, and to map the courses that may lead toward control of costs. One that looks possible is the effort now being made to infuse some competition into the health care industry through organized systems of care, known as HMOs.

Health maintenance organizations, especially the fee-for-service variety known as IPAs (individual practice associations), have been a particular interest of the Center for Industry and Health Care, where a national data base on IPA performance is being established with the aid of the Robert Wood Johnson Foundation. The Center's identity with HMOs, combined with its focus on industry and health care, has afforded us unusual access to nascent corporate thinking on the pros and cons of HMO sponsorship. We are grateful for these opportunities, and for the insights industry people have shared with us. This series draws heavily on that experience.

Previous volumes in the series have touched on HMOs, but none with the comprehensiveness attempted here. The first volume, in providing an overview and road map for the series as a whole, briefly discussed the possibility of industry's offering the HMO option as a modification to the benefit package, or sponsoring HMO development as an alternative delivery system. The second volume described a range of corporate innovations, HMO sponsorship among them. The third volume, a collection of papers on industry's changing role in the delivery of health care, included descriptions of two industry-sparked HMOs, written by their corporate sponsors. The fourth discussed industry's role in communicating information about health services generally and in transmitting to employee groups the marketing messages of HMOs seeking enrollees.

The point of departure for the more comprehensive treatment of HMOs in this fifth volume of the series is Secretary Califano's National HMO Conference, convened for business and labor leaders on March 10, 1978 by the Department of Health, Education, and Welfare. The journey comes full circle six months later with a panel discussion of corporate HMO activities, part of the "National Conference and Workshop on the IPA-HMO," held on September 15, 1978 in Aspen, Colorado by the Rocky Mountain Health Maintenance Organization, Inc. In between, the IPA-HMO concept was subject to a thorough review by the Massachusetts Division of Insurance during hearings on the Bay State Health Care Foundation's application for an HMO license. Summaries of these three events appear as appendices of the monograph; the text of chapter 3 draws on yet another conference: "Industry and HMOs in Massachusetts," a follow-up of the March 10 HEW conference, co-sponsored in April by the Center for Industry and Health Care of Boston University and the Massachusetts Society of Internal Medicine.

To the organizers of the conferences we owe a debt of gratitude, in particular to Edmond E. Charrette, M.D., immediate past president of the Massachusetts Society of Internal Medicine and Michael J. Weber, executive director of the Rocky Mountain Health Maintenance Organization, Inc. For a critical review of a draft of the book we are indebted to Jacob J. Spies, vice president, Employers Insurance of Wausau. As usual, Willis B. Goldbeck was extremely helpful, both for his own specific suggestions on the manuscript and on behalf of the Washington Business Group on Health, whose member corporations have been a major source of information and advice.

Although an artifact, the six-month period that this volume spans was a time of unusual ferment. Not only were there conferences and hearings, but several important HMO studies were published in professional journals during this period, and many corporate executives began in earnest to ask whether and how industry should promote the growth of HMOs. Their search for answers raises policy issues that bridge the separation between the series' two audiences—one in industry, the other in health care.

Preserving the timeliness of the material encompassed in the six-month cycle was an overriding objective which required making some compromises. For example, as we write this preface, the September panel discussion for appendix III has not yet taken place; it will be added to the book in production. This monograph, although far from exhaustive, is designed to be an up-to-date progress report on the state of HMO development and industry's possible role therein.

Boston, August 1978   Richard H. Egdahl

Diana Chapman Walsh

Contents

What Can Industry Do for HMOs and HMOs for Industry?

Diana Chapman Walsh

Any doubts that may have lingered about the place of health care costs on the national agenda were officially laid to rest by President Carter's cost-conscious national health insurance principles, outlined in late July 1978 by Secretary of Health, Education, and Welfare, Joseph Califano.[1] Costs now stand out as the most immediate problem of national health policy. Nearly all comprehensive cost control schemes accord the health maintenance organization a significant role, justified on both theoretical and practical grounds. And most proponents of health maintenance organizations are now looking to private industry as a source of leadership and support. This is a relatively new development and could bring dramatic results, should industry accept the challenge. The purpose of this book, the fifth in the Springer Series on Industry and Health Care, is to unravel that challenge to industry and examine its implications, from the perspectives of both industry and the health care system.

HMOs and Health Care Costs

Competition is the core concept around which wind the theoretical threads of the case for HMOs.[2-4] Economists blame lack of economic competition for escalating costs and theorize that rising health care costs bespeak incentives gone awry—an insurance system that underwrites care for "consumers" who need not or cannot "shop" for a sound medical buy from "providers" who can generate demand for services, recover costs, and "optimize" incomes. Prepaid health plans (HMOs) emerge from this analysis as a logical mechanism for setting the incentives right and injecting competition into the health care system. HMOs circumscribe within a fixed budget the traditional open-ended relationship between providers, patients, and payers. Providers contract to deliver a specified package of services to a defined population for a fixed premium, established on the basis of actuarial projections. The consumer, in deciding to enroll, also locks himself in. He now has to pay out-of-pocket should he choose to go outside of the HMO for a health care service available through the plan. With the sky no longer the limit on health care spending in this closed financial system, incentives can be introduced to encourage providers and consumers to conserve finite resources.

HMO proponents contend that if several such plans operate within a single geographical area, they will become accountable for their performance to a degree unknown in the traditional health care system. Each HMO will be forced to compete for members (patients) on the basis of product and price. The self-discipline that is likely to result is illustrated by the Minneapolis experience, described in chapter 3, case 6. Chapter 5 posits that market-oriented approaches stand the best chance of permanently and satisfactorily solving the problem of rising health care costs.

The practical rationale for prepaid health plans is their developing record. A few prototypes emerged well before the turn of the century. Their first spurt of growth occurred in the 1930s; in the 1970s they became an instrument of national health policy,[5] based on persuasive evidence of their capacity under the right circumstances to provide medical care at lower cost than the traditional unstructured system. A few studies have shown that successful mature plans, such as Kaiser Permanente in California (see chapter 3, case 1) have cut costs by 10 to 40 percent. Many more studies indicate that various types of prepaid plans make considerably less use of the hospital, with no evidence of compromised quality as compared to the traditional system.[6] Since hospital costs account for a major share of health care costs, this finding explains most of the demonstrated savings of the well established plans and suggests that prepaid plans generally should have significant potential for controlling costs by minimizing their dependence on expensive inpatient services.

Despite their popularity in political circles, prepaid health plans have taken hold less rapidly than it was hoped they would when, in 1971, their development was espoused as national policy.[7] About 170 plans now enroll under seven million members—only about 3 percent of the U. S. population.[8] (Figure 1) Many plans were started during the early 1970s, and that growth has continued. Between 1976 and 1977, the number of operating HMOs increased by almost 15 percent.[9] Still, the older plans account for almost three-quarters of

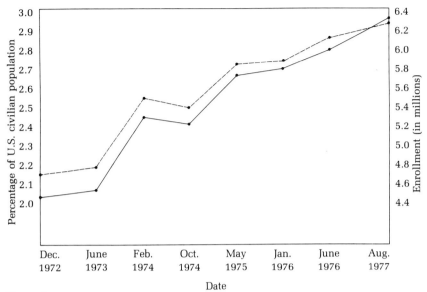

Figure 1

Enrollment in HMOs, 1972–1977. (——) = Number of members; (– – –) = Percentage of U.S. civilian population. *Sources:*

HMO Enrollment:
1. U.S. Department of Health, Education, and Welfare, Office of the Assistant Secretary for Health, Office of Health Maintenance Organizations. Program Status Reports (December 1972; June 1973; February 1974; October 1974; May 1975; and December 1976), Rockville, Maryland.
2. Group Health Association of America. *National HMO Census Survey 1977.* Washington, D.C.

U.S. Civilian Population:
1. *The Handbook of Basic Economic Statistics*, Vol. 32, Nos. 1 and 4 (January and April 1978). Economic Statistics Bureau, Washington, D.C.
2. *Current Population Reports: Population Estimates and Projections.* U.S. Department of Commerce, Series P-25, No. 504, August 1973.

total HMO enrollment, and the rate of increase in membership has fallen short of expectations. There are various explanations for the disappointing growth rate. High on the list is the undeniable fact that HMOs are difficult to start because they necessitate major changes in the behavior of physicians and patients. An important question for industry, then, is when is the effort justified, and this is a question that several large industrial firms are now investigating.

Industry and HMOs

The question splits into two. First, what can HMOs do for industry, to ease the financial burden of paying for employees' health care without taking away benefits or compromising the quality of care? Second, what can industry do for the HMO "movement," to realign the incentives in health care, foster competition, and thereby build private sector solutions to the dilemma of rising costs? An objective of this monograph, and indeed of the entire Series on Industry and Health Care, is to stimulate a dialogue on this two-part question. Underlying the series is the assumption that industry can act as an important agent of change in the health care system over the next several years. One critical test of that assumption will occur in the HMO arena.

Industry's involvement with prepaid health care antedates the "HMO movement," as chapter 3 attests. From the outset, architects of the movement have viewed employee groups as a major source of potential HMO members. The fourth volume of this series[10] described the dual-choice provision of the 1973 Health Maintenance Organization Act,[11] and the challenge of marketing HMOs to employee groups accustomed to traditional third-party health insurance.

The government has now moved beyond the dual-choice requirement and has called on industry to do more for HMOs than merely serve as a hospitable but relatively passive conduit of marketing information to employees. That call to action was symbolized by Secretary Califano's HMO Conference, described in appendix I. It seemed to reflect the hope that industry might strengthen the mildly anemic HMO movement if large corporations decide to use their prestige and resources to sponsor, or at least spark, the development of HMOs for their employees. This is HEW's answer to the second half of the two-part question of the mutual interests between industry and HMOs. Less clear, at this juncture, is industry's answer to the first. The extent to which corporations will choose to become actively involved in HMO sponsorship remains clouded. Like any lasting partnership, the association between industry and HMOs will work well only if it involves an identifiable quid pro quo. As chapter 2 indicates, several firms are now engaged in the process of assessing what they would stand to gain or risk in sponsoring their own HMOs.

The first and highest hurdle they encounter is how to pin down basic definitions: what, exactly, is this thing they might sponsor and where are the applicable models? Even the generic term HMO is often called into question on grounds that prepaid plans really do not maintain health but rather introduce management rigors. As the acronyms are peeled away, it seems there are almost as many layers of different HMO variants as there are individual prepaid plans. Shifting definitional sands under the HMO movement make for unstable terrain. Federal qualification means one thing, and brings its own baggage of lables and acronyms. But some plans never see the need to seek qualification as chapter 3 attests, and even the largest and most famous—the Kaiser plans—only recently took the trouble to become federally qualified. Definitional obscurity confounds the descriptive facts—how many HMOs exist, how many people they serve, and at what rate they are growing. Figure 1 represents our best effort at piecing together a trend line, but for nearly every number we settled on, others seemed equally plausible.

The conceptual framework we use throughout this book, because of its relative simplicity and convenience, divides HMOs into two broad categories reflecting the way they organize and pay participating physicians: "closed-panel" salaried group plans and "open-panel" fee-for-service plans. The two major types subdivide into the various other models described in chapter 3 and are now also beginning to evolve into hybrid forms, seeking to preserve the best of both species.

Chapter 3 describes these major HMO types, illustrated with case descriptions, defines basic concepts, and outlines a broad approach for assessing alternative models in the context of community health resources available to the sponsoring company. Chapter 4 identifies the primary legal hurdles and examines what it may take to clear them.

Chapter 5 identifies salient issues for the future, implicitly making the point that several basic questions about HMO potential still lack optimal or even satisfactory answers. The ideas of four corporate executives bent on finding answers that are, if not optimal, at least appropriate for presentation to top management as part of a recommended course of action, is the focus of appendix III.

According to remarks made at a recent Conference Board meeting,[12] the 1973 Health Maintenance Organization Act has set "the stage for the reorganization of the health care delivery system in the United States." If the stage is in fact set, the script is still in flux. New actors are being recruited to sponsor and promote HMOs, others are wandering off, and the shifting cast of characters makes for a volatile production. Industry now has the option of assuming whatever role it finds most promising for its many constituents. In doing so, of course, industry could inadvertently—or quite deliberately—rewrite the script entirely.

NOTES

1. Philip Shabecoff, "President Outlines His Plan on Health; Focus on Economics," *New York Times* (July 20, 1978): 1.

2. Warren Greenberg, ed., *Competition in the Health Care Sector: Present, Past, and Future* (Washington, D.C.: Federal Trade Commission, Bureau of Economics, March 1978).

3. Alain C. Enthoven, "Consumer-Choice Health Plan," *New England Journal of Medicine 298* (March 23, March 30, 1978): 650–658, 709–720.

4. Clark C. Havighurst, "Controlling Health Care Costs: Strengthening the Private Sector's Hand," *Journal of Health Politics, Policy, and Law 1* (1977): 291–498.

5. Paul M. Ellwood, Jr., *et al.*, "Health Maintenance Strategy," *Medical Care 9* (1971): 291–298.

6. Harold S. Luft, "How Do Health Maintenance Organizations Achieve Their Savings?" *New England Journal of Medicine 298* (June 15, 1978): 1336–1343.

7. Paul Starr, "The Undelivered Health System," *The Public Interest 42* (1976): 68–85.

8. Lawrence Meyer, "Health Plans Grew in Seven Years But Not As Much As Expected," *Washington Post* (January 3, 1978): 7a.

9. Metropolitan Life Insurance Co., "Health Maintenance Organizations (HMOs)," *Statistical Bulletin* (April–June 1978): 5–6.

10. Richard H. Egdahl and Diana Chapman Walsh, eds., *Health Services and Health Hazards: The Employee's Need to Know*, Springer Series on Industry and Health Care, No. 4 (New York: Springer-Verlag, 1978).

11. P. L. 93-222 (42 U.S.C. 300e Supp. IV, 1974).

12. David A. Weeks, ed., *Rethinking Employee Benefit Assumptions* (New York: The Conference Board, 1978): p. 12.

Defining Corporate Strategies and Goals

Diana Chapman Walsh

Prompted by concern over the accelerating costs of employee health benefits, executives in scores of large corporations are wondering whether they might gain more efficient management of those dollars by sponsoring one or more HMOs for employees of the firm and their dependents. Some firms are actively studying the option on the way to an immediate decision. With the notable exceptions, described in chapter 3, of Kaiser Industries, R. J. Reynolds Corporation, and coalitions of employers in Minneapolis and greater Philadelphia, most such firms are at present grappling with first- or second-order issues of feasibility, desirability, and cost effectiveness. The more practical issues of implementation are still a year or two down the road, should the decision be made to sponsor an HMO. These firms are approaching the analysis deliberately and with as much objectivity as they can muster. But they are also mindful that the day will soon come when "our objectivity will have to give way to a concrete recommendation to our executive committee."

In consultations over the past year or two with representatives of a dozen or more corporations assessing HMOs, we have developed a feel for how the decision is being approached. The firms are creating the process as they go along. There is no rational template or master plan, and only a few available publications have direct pertinence to the decision-making process per se. For example, the federal government published an *HMO Feasibility Study Guide*[1] in 1974. In a 1973 *Harvard Business Review* article, Dr. Paul Ellwood and Michael Herbert of InterStudy encouraged business to take its own look at HMO sponsorship and suggested some criteria to use.[2] Under the aegis of the National Chamber Foundation, InterStudy is now developing more specific guidelines for businesses interested in taking a closer look.[3,4]

To some extent the HMO consideration is a judgment of the sort that industry routinely makes. It involves such generic business principles as clarifying objectives to reflect the firm's philosophy, strengths, and weaknesses; developing an adequate data set from which to construct realistic pictures of the firm's situation compared with others in similar circumstances; and projecting alternative scenarios for the future that take adequate account of the firm's internal needs and its relations with its "environment," as well as its competitive position in national and world markets.

Substance rather than process is usually where difficulties arise. Information is often sketchy on the specifics of the firm's current health costs and on the "track records" of the newer forms of HMO and how they might perform in widely varying industrial settings. After pressing hard the issue of track records of fee-for-service HMOs, one benefits manager summarized the problem succinctly:

> I think what I'm hearing you say is that these creatures are promising fillies—that is, for the most part, they don't yet have solid track records, in part because they are still evolving.

The response is yes, successive generations of fee-for-service HMOs are applying progressively more sophisticated and rigorous HMO principles to the conventional methods of delivering personal health services. The latest renditions are only a few months old—too little time has elapsed to evaluate their capabilities. The future shape they may take will depend in large part on how actively industry chooses to become involved in the process of their creation. For reasons explored in chapter 3, fee-for-service HMOs provide greater flexibility and may be easier to start than classic closed panel plans. Because they less profoundly disrupt traditional patterns of behavior, fee-for-service HMOs usually enroll larger proportions of the employee groups they approach than do salaried plans. As a result, even if the per-member cost of the plan is somewhat higher, the wider employee participation may mean greater management impact for the employer.

To set the stage for the description of HMOs contained in chapter 3, this chapter extracts the essence of some discussions we have had with corporate people looking at HMO sponsorship and pieces together a composite picture of the process that seems to be unfolding and the concerns that seem to surface repeatedly in different settings and circumstances in large industrial firms across the country. Because their thinking is in the formative stage. few of the

individuals consulted are in a position to "go public" with their plans. Therefore, the comments that we quote, although genuine, are unavailable for at-
tribution. They are supplemented, however, by the Aspen, Colorado panel
discussion, summarized in appendix III, where the participants did speak for
the record. The purpose of this chapter and the accompanying appendix is to
bring major issues into focus and disseminate the thoughts of corporate executives who have progressed rather far in the process of analyzing corporate
sponsorship of HMOs.

Organizational Patterns and Beginning Steps

The task may fall to the risk manager, the director of employee benefits,
the corporate medical director, the corporate health planner, or sometimes to
someone farther afield. Typically, the individual is working alone or as part of a
very small task force assigned to study the problem of the rising costs of the
employee health benefit and to propose solutions. The origins and specific
nature of their mandates and objectives vary. At one extreme is the firm looking
for ways to "get things going more effectively in the community in order to
move health services out of the house and concentrate on the things we do
well." The other extreme is represented by the company hoping to expand its
clinical facilities, bring the HMO's laboratory testing in-house, and develop
close relationships with HMO physicians in the areas of workmen's compensation and occupational health screening, as well as personal health services.

Corporate structure, management philosophy, and interpersonal dynam-
ics within the organization also vary, along with the history of each company, its product lines, economic and geographic environments, and work
force. These can be decisive factors, of course, but they elude meaningful
generalizations. Still, there are discernable patterns. Issues of power and control within the corporation lie close to the surface, and the fate of a project may
hang in the delicate balance between the medical, benefits, finance, and industrial relations divisions. Firms pursuing the analysis of HMOs most aggressively have relieved one or two people of some—occasionally all—of their
routine duties for a period of time to tackle the problem, but more often it is an
added burden on an already heavy work load. The amount of time available to
spend on the project may be an index of the degree of corporate commitment to
finding a solution, and in some cases the first challenge is to arouse enough
concern at high levels to buy some time to study the problem. Corporate
commitment is nearly always cited as a sine qua non. Even those with strong
sanction from top management often worry about the lack of appreciation up
and down the management line for the problem of health care costs, and place
high on their list of priorities the need to convince management in both the
home office and the field of the need for concerted efforts to bring these costs
under control.

In most of the cases in our initial sampling, the first step of securing a
mandate has already been taken and a senior executive officer or executive
committee has been "charged up" about the problem of rising health care costs.
Frequently, this has been accomplished by projecting cost increases over the
next five or ten years and demonstrating their impact. One firm with annual

sales of around $3 billion estimates that if past trends continue over the next ten years, the firm could spend a total of $2.5 billion on health benefits. "That's a number," the benefits manager says, "that makes management sit up and listen."

Typically, the second step has also been taken: a list of possible cost containment strategies has been compiled and assessed from the perspective of the firm. One benefits manager with an engineering background described a vision he once had of developing a cost containment strategy in health much as a firm might approach a multimillion dollar engineering project, with decisions specified in sequence and contingencies covered systematically. Now he dismisses the idea as an unrealistic goal. Others make similar comments:

> Over a year ago we put together a list from which we thought rather naively we would find success stories we could simply replicate. We find now that there are very few success stories just ripe for replication, although there are claimed successes for HMOs and that's why we're now focusing on them.

Behind that word "claimed" are hours of practical experiences with HMOs. Invariably, the corporate task force includes someone well versed in HMO lore. The firm typically belongs to one or more organizations (like the Washington Business Group on Health and the National Association of Employers on HMOs), subscribes to specialized periodicals (like Business Insurance and the Spencer publications), and sends representatives to meetings (like those summarized in this volume) that cover HMOs in excruciating detail. These firms, in short, approach HMOs with their eyes open, and usually with a certain amount of skepticism based on disappointing enrollment experiences or other concerns about the financial viability of particular plans—concerns that are rarely unfounded but that tend to derive chiefly from the company's own experience, which may be dated or incomplete, and from anecdotal evidence that may not be relevant to the company's location or situation.

The countervailing concern is the slope of the cost curve and the apparent ineffectiveness of incremental approaches to cost containment. The list of possible programs seems to be endless and diffuse. For example, having recently shepherded six new cost containment projects through the corporate executive committee, the benefit department of one large Eastern company faces a list of twenty-nine additional possibilities awaiting careful analysis. In this milieu the HMO's relative comprehensiveness is a major virtue. As a closed management system with fixed dollars, it seems to incorporate many of the other discrete cost control measures on the master list. To a beleaguered benefits manager, this has intuitive appeal; the question is how to get there from here.

Savings Potential in an HMO: The First Cut and a Second Look

The corporate analyst who looks closely at the successes claimed for HMOs finds few specific or recent assertions about costs. Instead, the most persistent claim on behalf of HMOs is that they can reduce the hospitalization rate to 500 or so days per 1,000 enrollees. A large corporation can easily convert this statistic into theoretical savings—and they are consequential. For example, the personnel director of a multibillion dollar industrial firm stated it this way in a memorandum to top management:

> It may be possible in the future to reduce our hospital utilization rate from over 1,000 days per 1,000 employees and dependents to around 500 days per 1,000, with a potential savings of more than $15 million per year . . . by introducing a company-related health maintenance organization to reduce hospital utilization with no sacrifice in the quality of care.

Those who start with this calculation recognize it as the roughest of first cuts and carefully point out that a front-end investment must be amortized before realizing savings. Even more important, at least six implicit assumptions need close examination:

1. Is the figure for the firm's current hospital days per 1,000 employees and dependents reasonably accurate?

2. Is the population generating those days roughly comparable to populations served by the types of HMOs in the 500-days-per-1,000-enrollees range that the firm would consider sponsoring?

3. Will a substantial proportion of employees elect to join the HMO? (Actually, the computation assumes that all will belong to the HMO, which is an unrealistic expectation if the employees are given a real option.)

4. Will the hospital days averted translate into dollar savings and not simply into increased ambulatory care, ancillary services, or administrative and overhead costs, spread over fewer days?

5. Will the dollars saved return to—or not leave—the corporation's balance sheet, or at least be reflected as a reduction in the employee's out-of-pocket expenses?

6. Will the HMO prove feasible from the standpoint of medical politics, corporate policies, regulatory hurdles, and labor relations?

Data Deficiencies: Approximations and Proxies

Whether undertaken in-house or by an outside consulting firm, analysis of these assumptions requires a solid data base. "Denominator data" are needed to describe the population at issue ("at risk" in public health parlance) and "numerator data" to delineate reasonable expectations of HMO performance. In several instances, gathering essential denominator data on the current situation in employee health benefits is taxing the very limits of the firms' data collection capabilities and those of its insurance carrier. To define the population at risk fairly precisely, the employer needs a zip code distribution of employees' residences, information on the average number of dependents covered in family contracts, and age distribution by sex (ideally encompassing both employees and dependents, although we find few firms with such specific dependent data.) A geographical breakdown of salary and hourly status and/or union and nonunion status could be useful if the firm might consider offering the plan initially only to one of these groups.

In corporations where personnel data maintenance is not a centralized function, some divisions may be able to provide this information easily while others cannot. Information on dependents tends to become outdated quickly; it is often recorded on manual enrollment cards with the insurance carrier (sometimes for life insurance, rather than for health), or on pre-employment forms stored somewhere in cardboard cartons, still uncoded and unlikely ever to be updated. Where denominator data are lacking, the assessment has to proceed on the basis of reasonable assumptions and best guesses.

Unless the firm directly administers its own health care claims, maintaining data on employee utilization of the health benefit is normally the responsibility of the health insurance carrier. In fact, the drift in some firms towards self-insurance (the subject of number six of this series, currently in press) seems in large part to reflect dissatisfaction with the carrier's performance in the realm of data maintenance. Although fairly widespread, criticism of carrier data reporting to major policyholders is a recent phenomenon, usually tempered with the recognition that the "rules" are subtly changing. As one benefits manager observed:

> Until very recently, there was no management pressure nor a perceived management payoff to make the investment it would take to set up a decent system for tracking absenteeism and the use of the health benefit. The insurance companies have presumably been spinning out data for years and nobody has ever bothered to look at it. Now, suddenly, there is a great clamor for data, and everyone's waking up to the fact that the information the carriers have been collecting is not terribly helpful.

Another corporation—one of the world's largest—is studying the advisability of developing this data capacity internally, to the tune of about $1 million: "With our $750 million investment every year," the corporate medical director says, "we buy a lot of health care. But we really don't know what we are buying." A senior financial officer concurs:

> I don't know if we have a problem, but that in itself represents a problem. I see rules of thumb abounding on cost control, but I don't even know for certain how much of our money is going to hospital inpatient services as opposed to ambulatory care or for care of employees as distinct from dependents. We have drifted piecemeal into full service coverage and now we need cost control and for that we need data—on incidences and durations of medical episodes by diagnosis, age, sex, and geographical location. We need trend analyses and we need a way to compare our experiences to those of other relevant populations and among matched populations with different benefit plan designs. And we're willing to pay for that base-line data set.

The paramount reason there has been no demand for this base-line data until recently is that, traditionally, fair and expeditious processing of claims has been the overriding goal in managing an employee health benefit. Record-keeping practices have reflected this claims orientation. The transactions most faithfully counted are claims filed and bills processed—measures which neither necessarily nor even usually bear a one-to-one correspondence with significant medical encounters. One hospital admission may produce one or several billings, and carrier data systems have tended to overlook this distinction. On policies with a deductible, some or all of the medical care purchased by the employee may never be recorded because the employee has not reached the threshhold where the policy would begin paying and has forgotten to report out-of-pocket expenditures, or because the carrier's data system is claims-rather than patient-oriented and records only those claims actually paid.

Large firms with plants or offices spread across the country sometimes pay premiums on a national rate which does not reflect regional differences. For example, Oregon employees may be indirectly (if the employer pays the premium) and unwittingly subsidizing the care of employees based in Massachusetts. Carriers usually make use of "loss ratios," which show these differences in gross terms, but again these data tend to be oriented to claims and not to utilization rates for specific services. In fact, anomalies in the loss ratios in different parts of the country, unexplained by differences in health status, are frequently among the initial concerns prompting a firm to consider a different way to manage the health care dollar. One of the anticipated by-products of HMO sponsorship is better data on which to base future decisions.

The Current Benefit Package and Management–Labor Relations

The existing benefit package—its financing and administration, and especially its scope—to some extent influences the potential effectiveness of a corporate-sponsored HMO in containing the firm's own costs. The present arrangement forms the bench mark against which anticipated HMO performance can be calibrated. Where evidence can be found of "slack" in the current financing and administration of the plan or in the community medical care system embracing it (for example, high utilization rates for hospitalization or particular types of elective surgery, steep administrative costs, poor coordination of benefits, excess hospital beds, or high physician fees), it stands to reason that the HMO will have a running start on cost savings. If, to the contrary, a full panoply of cost control measures already exists (such as utilization review, second surgical opinion, good hospital bed control, reasonable professional fees, coordination of benefits, tight financing arrangements with the carrier through a minimum premium plan, administrative-services-only agreement, or full self-insurance), the HMO's short-term savings may be more modest.

In the context of the existing package there is, moreover, a kind of "Catch 22." If the medical benefit is already comprehensive and fully financed by the employer, the most optimistic of HMO marketers may foresee difficulty in persuading employees that their interests are served by enrolling in the HMO. However dramatic the estimates of per-employee cost savings potential in the HMO, a company will not save money if employees will not join. In situations such as this, other employee incentives must be identified, perhaps better access to care without the bother of filing claims forms, and "one-stop shopping" for comprehensive medical care.

Marketing should surely be simpler where the current package is less liberal from the employee's perspective, which usually means that the employee is responsible for deductibles and co-payment on routine physician services. The HMO must eliminate or substantially reduce these expenses in order to give the physicians the latitude they need to contain costs. In so doing, the plan will appeal to the employee as an expanded benefit capable of reducing out-of-pocket expenditures for health care. But here is the catch: if the employer currently pays the full premium and expects to continue doing so for the firm's HMO, then some portion of the savings the firm could realize through the HMO will be lost in the shift away from cost sharing with employees for their routine ambulatory care. The cost differential can be effectively offset by sharing the premium cost with employees in the HMO if the HMO's benefit package is considerably broader, and if current out-of-pocket expenditures can be identified for the employee. He is, after all, used to contributing to his health care costs.

Labor relations underlie the "Catch 22," since they constrain the employer's decision on the financing of the HMO benefit. Always a salient factor, the union situation varies widely, from the unusual case in which the benefits manager can say:

We have no union; we just do what we think makes sense,

to the other extreme, represented by a medium-sized firm (annual sales of $600 million) with 7,000 employees, seven major unions, nine different benefit packages, plus a corporate plan. The annual rate of cost increase is over 15 percent, and most of the plans are entirely noncontributory. The firm's assistant treasurer worries:

> *From where I sit this is an area I don't think we manage effectively. But we're prisoners of our past. We've acceded to union demands year after year without any thought to the long-range implications. I'm really not convinced that there's any way we can turn back now.*

The majority of firms fall between these two extremes, but even those with unusually wide latitude in their labor relations would sooner compromise in terms of cost containment than jeopardize a tranquil labor situation. Quite apart from any marketing implications, few firms seem ready to institute an employer-sponsored HMO without reasonable assurance that doing so would enhance, or at least not threaten, the firm's employee relations and its bargaining posture with its unions.

The Physician–Patient Relationship and the Tightrope of Medical Politics

Concerns about employee reactions and a reluctance to interfere with employee relationships with physicians have pointed several firms in the direction of the fee-for-service HMO, either in conjunction with or instead of the traditional closed panel model. A senior executive of an insurance carrier re-examining its HMO stance said this:

> If we could do only one type of HMO we would do an IPA. I am a trustee of my community hospital and I watched the fur fly when the medical staff there was approached by a closed panel HMO looking for a suburban hospital base. Closed panel plans are going to recreate that scene over and over again in hospital after hospital. It's going to be a slow painful process.

In a different corporation, the benefits manager paints a similar picture:

> We've had several meetings with the physicians in town and they've brought home to us the traumatic shock you might have to force on a community to bring an HMO into being. We think an IPA will lead to fewer employee relations problems that would tend to spin off of physician hostility. If it can influence the cost curve, an IPA might work where a closed panel would not.

Meetings with local physicians—to seek their cooperation in helping to contain costs, to gauge the intensity of opposition to HMOs, or to identify potential leadership should an HMO project be launched—have already been held by nearly all the corporations in our sample. Occasionally, the president or chief executive officer has presided. Without fail, the organizers of such meetings have alerted top management in advance, to anticipate the likelihood that word of it would spread quickly through personal relationships between physicians and officers in the firm. One reason middle managers would prefer to avoid stirring up physician antipathy is brought into sharp focus by a comment made by one benefits manager. The specific circumstances vary from company to company but the general situation is virtually universal:

> My boss' boss recently underwent successful open-heart surgery. You can be sure that I won't win points with him by going around knocking doctors.

Particularly in a mid-sized or smaller city, where top managers in large corporations tend to move in the same social circles as does the medical establishment, middle managers confronting cost escalation in health are acutely sensitive to "the diverse and disparate interests in a corporation that have to be brought along on this." This issue of medical politics worries them most of all.

> As laymen, we have a serious lack of understanding of how the physician community really operates. The most articulate doctor

in town and probably the most vociferous is twenty years behind the times. Though he's held several positions of leadership in the medical community, we're told he doesn't speak for the profession—that no one does. But where, then, do we find progressive physician leadership? We're by far the largest employer in town but we'll get nowhere without a critical mass of physician support.

This corporation is trying to enlist a few physician leaders—progressives who accept the need for cost control and want to participate in building future health care systems. They can help organize a select physician group to set the ground rules for the fee-for-service HMO as a management system. This process should be guided by the HMO principles elaborated in chapter 3, including rigorous utilization review based on a good data system, sharing of financial risk by participating physicians, effective management, marketing, and perhaps some membership selection to ensure that at least those physicians with demonstrably wasteful practice patterns are excluded from the plan. On this last principle, opinion is divided. If physicians known to be "overutilizers" are excluded from membership in the fee-for-service HMO, the plan is likely to have an easier time holding down its costs. But it may have less impact on community-wide costs than it could have by training its peer review spotlight on the physicians with the most costly practice patterns. Where the scales will tip for a given corporation will depend on its particular objectives in sponsoring the HMO.

For all their diffidence about physician sensitivities and politics, corporate executives know they have unusual potential leverage within the health care system, as major purchasers of care. Some are coming close to the point where they are ready to use that leverage:

It's very clear that there will have to be some powerful motivation before doctors will change their ways. You've called it fear. It's really a combination of economic and professional self-interest, I guess. But in the real world, where we think we are, if we have to appeal to those motives among physicians then we will. I don't care if we have an IPA; I do care about the slope of that cost curve.

Geography: Concentration and Clout

Given a choice of location, it may be more comfortable and safer to begin in the firm's own backyard; that is, near corporate headquarters. For many firms, but by no means all, the backyard beginning makes sense also from the standpoint of concentration of employees and potential "clout" in the community. Also, the project will be easier to implement and monitor in the place where it found its original impetus. On the other hand, the community influence represented in corporate headquarters is exercised within an intricate web of professional and personal ties. Corporate executives sit on the boards of local hospitals, other health agencies, and insurance companies, and these interlocking directorates confound the interactions between the firm and the health provider community. The complexity of these organizational and social relationships increases the inherent political sensitivities.

Several firms have discussed starting with the headquarters town on a pilot basis and later, when the HMO model is fully developed and "debugged," transferring it to other areas, where large concentrations of employees live and work. Depending on the size and spread of the firm, the possibilities range from one or two sites to twelve, fifteen, or perhaps many more:

> We're interested in places where we're enough of a presence to have an impact. It may be a cornfield where we're not that big by our own standards, but where we're the largest employer around.

In considering geography, the corporation must also resolve such issues as whether or not to collaborate with other firms in the same location and when to "surface publicly" in the planning process. Joining forces may enhance the project's aggregate influence but also tends to slow the process and dilute the control of any one participant. In volume 2 of this series Willis Goldbeck observed, "Although cooperation among employers is highly desirable, most companies have found that 'going it alone' at the start saves time and produces a faster return on investment."[5]

A corporation's decision to join forces with other corporations and community groups may be influenced by the relative priority given to "community service." One seldom discusses corporate sponsorship of HMOs without hearing some reference to community service and needs, but firms vary considerably in the importance accorded this goal.

The "Bottom Line" Is the Bottom Line . . .

Even those firms that weight community service heavily in their decision matrix arrive finally at the firm's bottom line. As one benefits manager put it:

> We don't want to sound cold or calculating, but if we find no economic justification, we're not interested. We have a community concern, and its a real one that will play a major part in our thinking. And we recognize that we may have to make a short-term investment to achieve better control over the next five to ten years. But if it looks like an IPA-HMO will reduce hospitalization without a reduction in cost—as some of the data suggest—then we have to ask ourselves, what's the justification for proceeding?

Others express similar opinions without the same willingness to wait for results:

> I want to see results in today's dollars. Five years ago the argument that we should merely address the slope of the cost curve might have been convincing, but with all the attention now being paid to health care costs, I'm not so sure. I believe a conservative estimate of the potential of one of these HMOs ought to show savings com-

*pared to the existing insurance arrangement. Without that I'll have
a tough time buying the idea myself, much less selling it across and
up the management line.*

Chapter 5 asserts that with hospital cost containment legislation apparently stalled in Congress, and with the strong emphasis on cost control contained in the Carter administration's national health insurance principles, it seems doubtful that costs are now coming under control. Even if they were, some kind of initiative on the part of industry would still be required, simply to manage more effectively the investment it is now making:

*To say that costs are high is not necessarily to say they're too high.
But once you recognize how much that health benefit is costing, you
then have to make darn sure that you understand where that money
is going. That means data. And that means controls of some kind. . . .
We're self-insured already and I'm convinced that our best hope now
is an HMO.*

Those firms interested in containing costs are careful to specify that they do not mean to compromise quality: "We're not looking to slash costs. We're willing to pay for quality," said one; another noted, "We're concerned now that spending more health care money on the employee's behalf may not represent an improvement." Still, for most corporations, the bottom line has particular salience, and if an HMO could cut the health benefit cost by only one-tenth, the effort would easily be justified. A 10 percent reduction in a health benefit bill of $45 million would add about $2.2 million to the bottom line of a typical firm, after taxes. Brought down to the bottom line, the issue translates to good management. The question, according to one vice president, boils down to this:

*Do we now have the framework within which our health care
dollars are being managed as efficiently, effectively, and eco-
nomically as they can be? If not, why not, and what do we need to
do?*

. . . Or Is It?

Pragmatic measures may win the day but philosophy often seems to finish a close second. The corporate executive rarely discusses health care costs without taking up the gauntlet that HEW Secretary Califano, the Council on Wage and Price Stability,[6] and others have thrown down for the private sector. Califano's call to action is summarized in appendix I. The response of one benefits manager is typical:

*The plate is overflowing and resources are thin. We are going to
have to face the question—do we think that the alternative to industry's really becoming actively involved in containing health care
costs can be so adverse that we really have no choice? What is the*

alternative? Drifting into more regulation and nationalization? If so, do we believe that people down the road will look back and say that was an awful thing for us to have let happen? I don't know. But that's the kind of question we're going to have to come to grips with over the next several months. Is this a problem like occupational cancer that simply demands our attention? Just how high on our corporate list of priorities should this problem be placed?

NOTES

1. U.S. Department of Health, Education, and Welfare, *HMO Feasibility Study Guide* (Washington, D.C.: Public Health Service, DHEW Publication No. HSA-74-1320, February 1974).

2. Paul M. Ellwood and Michael E. Herbert, "Health Care: Should Industry Buy It or Sell It?" *Harvard Business Review* (July-August 1973): 99–107.

3. John K. Tillotson and John C. Rosala, *A National Health Care Strategy: How Business Can Use Specific Techniques to Control Health Care Costs* (Washington, D.C.: prepared by InterStudy for the National Chamber Foundation, 1978).

4. Gerald B. Meier and Mary M. Hunter, *A National Health Care Strategy: How Business Can Stimulate a Competitive Health Care System* (Washington, D.C.: prepared by InterStudy for the National Chamber Foundation, 1978).

5. Willis B. Goldbeck, *A Business Perspective on Industry and Health Care*, Springer Series on Industry and Health Care, no. 2 (New York: Springer-Verlag, 1978), p. 49.

6. Executive Office of the President, Council on Wage and Price Stability, *The Complex Puzzle of Rising Health Care Costs: Can the Private Sector Fit It Together?* (Washington, D.C.: USGPO No. 053-003-00255-8, December 1976).

Identifying Available Options

Anthony J. Mahler and John Friedland

The Secretary's HMO Conference, summarized in appendix I, urged industry to become deeply involved in developing HMOs to help control the nation's health care costs. But aside from presenting a few case histories of company- or union-sponsored HMOs, the Conference fell short of providing specific plans for action. As a follow-up, the Center for Industry and Health Care and the Massachusetts Society for Internal Medicine sponsored a conference on industry and HMOs in Massachusetts. Drawing in part on comments by participants in the second conference, this chapter identifies various types of HMOs which a company can investigate once the decision has been made to pursue HMO development as an element in its strategy to contain health care costs. At this point in the process, an industry group must examine the health care system in its own community to find which of the possible HMO forms is appropriate for its specific situation. This chapter provides a background for that analysis.

The following discussion is based on particular definitions of certain key terms and on assumptions about the general functioning of an HMO. An HMO is an organization which guarantees delivery of a comprehensive, prepaid benefit package to a voluntarily enrolled population through an organized system of care. The term HMO is used here to mean both the plan as a whole and that specific part of the plan which performs the administrative duties, such as marketing, enrollment, claims processing, bookkeeping, and contracting for services.

HMOs can be classified in two broad categories, based on the way the "panel" of participating physicians is compensated. "Closed panel" or *salaried group HMOs* use group practices in which the physicians are paid salaries or on some other basis not directly related to the volume of services they provide, whereas "open panel" or *fee-for-service HMOs* are composed of physicians who receive fees for their services.[1] In the former category, the group practices devote some or all of their time to serving HMO members, while in the latter, physicians in various practice settings in a particular area serve HMO members as part of their practices. A third category, *direct capitation*, includes elements of the first two. The classification scheme used in this chapter is illustrated in figure 1. The different approaches to applying HMO concepts to combinations of existing providers in a community represent some of the more innovative efforts at HMO development. Federal law has recognized only three HMO structures: the Individual Practice Association (IPA) model, which is usually a fee-for-service HMO, and the staff and medical group models of the salaried group HMO.

The *physician component* comprises those physicians who agree to deliver a defined set of medical services to HMO members. The physician component may be a separate legal entity, such as a multispecialty group practice, or an IPA, in which case the legal entity will have some contractual relationship with the individual physicians. Where there is no legal entity, the individual physicians contract directly with the HMO.

The discussion which follows focuses on the physician component of HMOs, rather than on the hospital or administrative components. Since the physician controls diagnosis and treatment decisions—and thus costs—the key to cost control is involvement of the physician in the cost control process. Also, physician components vary widely from one type of HMO to another, often a decisive factor in how plans function.

The basic financial concept of an HMO is *capitation*, in which a predetermined amount of money is paid on a per-capita (i.e., per-member) basis for comprehensive health services. The HMO generally divides premium income into three separate funds. The *physician fund* is used to cover all payments to physicians and certain costs generated by physicians, such as outpatient diagnostic testing and referrals to specialists who are not part of the physician component. The *hospital fund* pays for services provided by hospitals, such as inpatient services and emergency care. The *administrative fund* is used not only to cover the HMO's direct administrative expenses, but also to purchase reinsurance policies and to build reserves. In terms of percent of premium, a rough breakdown of the relative size of these funds for a typical HMO might be 55 percent for the physician fund, 35 percent for the hospital fund, and 10 percent for the administrative fund.[2] Of course, there is considerable variation in these figures.

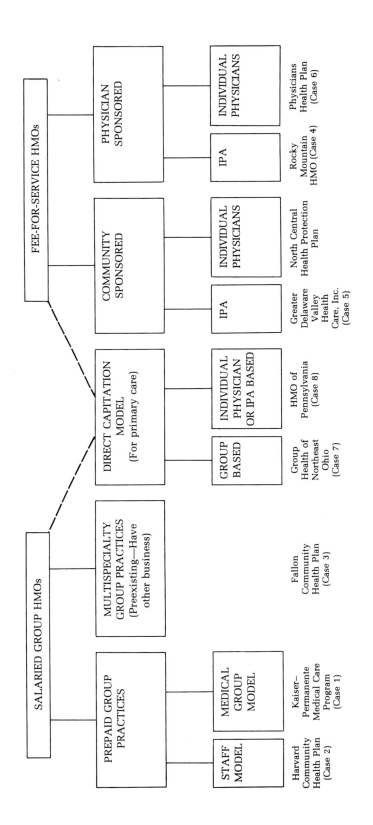

Figure 1
HMO classification.

Salaried Group HMOs: Roots in Prepaid Group Practices

The classic form of a salaried group HMO is a financing and medical organization called a prepaid group practice. One of the first was the Elk City, Oklahoma Farmers' Cooperative Clinic, established in the 1920s. Prepaid group practices are generally the best-known HMOs and the most significant in terms of enrollment. The six largest have some four million members, or 60 percent of all HMO enrollees, and include the Kaiser Foundation Health Plans, the Group Health Association of Washington, D.C., the Group Health Cooperative of Puget Sound, and the Ross-Loos HMO in Los Angeles. In fact, most subsequent HMO development is either modeled on, or a reaction to, the prepaid group practice form. Since it has frequently been discussed,[3] the concept and general structure of prepaid group practice is described only briefly in this book.

The physician component is a multispecialty group practice which has been developed specifically for the prepaid group practice. In the staff model the physicians are salaried employees of the HMO, whereas in the medical group model the group is a legal entity which contracts with the HMO. In the latter case, the group is paid out of the physician fund on a capitation basis. The group thus assumes some "risk" for medical services, since it has no recourse to patient members or the parent HMO organization if the group's expenditures exceed its income. Groups are usually organized as physician partnerships or professional corporations,[4] and the physicians must absorb deficits if they occur. The Permanente Medical Groups associated with the Kaiser Foundation Health Plans are an example of this structure (case 1).

The prepaid group practice structure has certain advantages for both physicians and patients. Physicians have the opportunity for greater peer interaction than is customary in solo practice, and since the group maintains central administrative services, physicians are relieved of many of the responsibilities unrelated to patient care which are generally part of private practice. The group also maintains its own laboratory and x-ray facilities to aid physicians in treating patients quickly and efficiently. The majority of referrals to other physicians can usually be made to other group physicians, using unit records which are based in a central location. These devices allow the group to offer HMO members services which are better coordinated than those usually provided in the traditional system of health care, and the central clinic facility gives the patient a single reference point for all medical services.

The prepaid group practice also encourages appropriate use of medical services. The financial structure removes the incentives to hospitalize which are present under traditional health insurance. Because many resources, such as diagnostic equipment and specialist consultants, are available at the clinic, physicians are less likely to refer patients outside the system. Furthermore, prepaid group practice emphasizes ambulatory, rather than inpatient, care with effective use of ancillary health personnel, such as nurse practitioners:

About 20 to 25 percent of our total visits to the Harvard Community Health Plan are to nurse practitioners and we're actually very proud of that because, quite frankly, we think it's just good medical care. Their productivity runs about half that of a physician, and their pay is approximately half. They have more of a tendency to use lab and x-ray or to refer to specialists than do the doctors themselves. So on balance, we don't look on them as cost-savers. We have a doctor and nurse who practice together; we integrate the two very tightly.

                                                                Gordon Moore*

The two most notable examples of company sponsorship of prepaid group practice HMOs are the Kaiser Industries[5] and R. J. Reynolds[6] plans. The Kaiser plans were originally set up in the 1930s and 1940s to serve Kaiser Industries' employees who could not get adequate medical care because of location, in the case of the workers on the Grand Coulee Dam, or wartime shortages of medical personnel, in the case of the San Francisco shipyard workers. The Kaiser plans were opened to the general public after the war, when employment at the shipyards plummeted, leaving a large clinical facility with a full medical staff. Similarly, R. J. Reynolds created the Winston-Salem Health Plan in 1975 to meet the needs of employees being transferred from New York to Winston-Salem and workers already located there, many of whom had been relying on local hospital emergency rooms for primary medical care.

The Kaiser plans have taken the integration of financing and medical care delivery a step further than most prepaid group practice HMOs by operating their own hospitals, usually as part of a complete facility which serves as both clinic and hospital for its members. This approach has provided even greater efficiencies by reducing duplication of laboratory and x-ray facilities and by matching the size of the facility as closely as possible to the needs of the enrolled population. The Kaiser system is thus able to serve its members with many fewer beds than are typically provided in the community at large. The Kaiser hospitals constitute a corporation, separate from the plan and physician group, and they operate on a prospectively fixed budget.

Organized labor has become a strong advocate of prepaid group practice HMOs, as reflected by George Meany's comments at Secretary Califano's HMO Conference (see appendix I). Labor unions, particularly the United Auto Workers and the AFL-CIO, have taken the lead in organizing several such plans, including the Rhode Island Group Health Association, the Metro Health Plan of Detroit, and the Community Health Plan of Cleveland.

Starting a prepaid group plan presents two major challenges beyond setting up a multispecialty group practice. The first is financial. The construction of a central clinical facility requires a minimum capital investment of approximately $2 million.[7] Also, expenses in the staff model are increased because of the need to maintain a salaried medical staff; the physicians must be paid whether or not there are members for them to serve. As the premium necessary to amortize these expenses rapidly would be prohibitively high for a new HMO, these plans can accumulate a large deficit before their membership exceeds the break-even point, which may take as long as five years. Break-even

*Medical Director, Cambridge Center, Harvard Community Health Plan; Associate Professor of Medicine, Harvard University.

CASE 1

Kaiser Permanente Medical Care Program

HMO Type: Salaried group (medical group model)

Location: Portions of: Northern California, Southern California, Oregon/Washington, Hawaii, Ohio, Colorado

Original sponsor(s): Corporate

Starting date: 1945

Service area population: 24,000,000

Enrollment: 3,500,000

Participating physicians: 3,400

In 1938, while preparing to start construction on the second phase of the Grand Coulee Dam in a remote area of Washington, the Henry J. Kaiser construction organization engaged Dr. Sidney Garfield to provide the workers and their families with a prepaid medical program, similar to one he had created in the Mojave Desert in 1933. The new program proved to be highly popular. Dr. Garfield's next assignment from Kaiser was to develop a medical care delivery system that would meet the needs of the wartime influx of workers to Kaiser's shipyards in the Portland/Vancouver and San Francisco areas and at a steel-mill east of Los Angeles. With the end of World War II and the marked curtailment of Kaiser's work force, the Kaiser Foundation Health Plan was opened to the general public in these areas.

The Kaiser-Permanente Medical Care Program has subsequently evolved to become the largest prepaid group practice operation, and, in fact, the largest nongovernmental provider of medical care, in the United States. With prepaid group practice plans in six regions, the overall program has twenty-eight hospitals, with approximately 5,900 beds, and seventy-three medical office facilities. Total revenues in 1977 exceeded one billion dollars.

In each region, the local nonprofit Kaiser Foundation Health Plan enters into contracts with subscriber groups and individuals to provide medical and hospital services. For legal reasons, the program has established separate health plans in the Colorado, Oregon, and Ohio regions, but the board structure of each of these plans is identical to that of the Kaiser Foundation Health Plan, Inc. which operates the plans in the other three regions. The Plan, in turn, enters into contracts with two other organizations, Kaiser Foundation Hospitals, and the regional Permanente Medical Group, to provide these services.

Kaiser Foundation Hospitals, a nonprofit corporation, owns and operates hospitals in each of the regions (except Colorado, where the plan uses community hospitals) as well as outpatient offices at the hospital sites. Kaiser Foundation Hospitals is compensated for its facilities and hospital services by the health plan according to a prospective budget that is based upon the former's "net financial requirements" (total costs, less nonplan revenues, plus provisions for the generation of cash to meet capital investment and debt service requirements). The boards of directors of Kaiser Foundation Hospitals and Kaiser Foundation Health Plan are identical.

An independent Permanente Medical Group exists in each region, and each is organized as either a professional partnership or a professional corporation. By contract with the local health plan, the local Permanente Medical Group agrees to provide all covered physician services, plus non-hospital services (laboratory and ancillary services, etc.) and personnel, in return for a negotiated monthly capitation payment. The physicians are salaried employees, partners (partner status is usually offered within three years of practice with the gruop) or shareholders of the group, with individual income levels set by the group. Group partners or shareholders also participate in an incentive bonus plan to reward efficiency, whereby they share in any surplus realized by the plan at year's end. The remainder of the surplus is provided to the hospitals for improvement or expansion of inpatient or unified inpatient/outpatient facilities, and/or retained by the health plan which is responsible for the financing of satellite outpatient facilities. The division of this surplus between the hospitals and the health plan is based on the needs of the regional program.

Each region has considerable autonomy, with the authority and responsibility for regional program decisions shared by the regional manager and regional medical director. The program also has a central office dealing with questions of program-wide concern, and a central policy-advisory body, the Kaiser-Permanente Committee, consisting of the regional managers and medical directors (chief executive officers of the Permanente Medical Groups) plus key central staff executives. Another program at the central level is Kaiser-Permanente Advisory Services, which advises outside organizations on issues related to prepaid, comprehensive, medical delivery programs.

In 1977 the Kaiser programs in all six regions were qualified under the federal HMO Act. While the programs are not themselves in need of federal loans or dual-choice leverage, many employers offering the Kaiser health plans urged them to become federally qualified so that the Kaiser option would satisfy the employer's obligation, under federal "dual choice" regulations, to offer one qualified group practice HMO to employees residing in areas served by such a plan. Hospital utilization in the regional health plans ranges from 391 to 491 days per 1,000 members per year.

Sources

Facts 1978 (Oakland, California: Kaiser Permanente Medical Care Program, Central Office Public Affairs Department, 1977).

Kaiser Foundation Medical Care Program, 1977 (Oakland, California: Kaiser Permanente Medical Care Program, 1977).

Scott Fleming, Senior Vice-President, Kaiser Foundation Health Plan, personal communication, August 1978.

Group Health Association of America. *National HMO Census Survey, 1977* (Washington, Group Health Association of America, 1977).

Jeffrey A. Prussin, "HMO's: Organizational and Financial Models (Part 3)," *Hospital Progress* (June 1974): 60–63.

Cecil C. Cutting, "Historical Development and Operating Concepts," in *The Kaiser-Permanente Medical Care Program: A Symposium*, Anne R. Somers, ed. (New York: The Commonwealth Fund, 1971), pp. 17–22.

Scott Fleming, "Anatomy of the Kaiser–Permanente Program," in *The Kaiser-Permanente Medical Care Program: A Symposium*, Anne R. Somers, ed. (New York: The Commonwealth Fund, 1971), pp. 23–32.

membership for a prepaid group practice HMO requires about 15,000 members or more, depending on the size of the clinical facility.[8]

Marketing is the second challenge. The prepaid group practice HMO must sell the new approach to medical service which it uses. Recent surveys show that the majority of people in the United States are satisfied with the way they currently receive medical care.[9] Consumers with traditional insurance coverage are free to choose any physician they want in the community and may also take the initiative in consulting a specialist. In contrast, members of a prepaid group practice HMO must receive medical care from the group's physicians at the central clinical facility. Also, the prepaid group practice HMO is more likely to use nurse practitioners and other ancillary personnel than are solo practice physicians. As a result, patients often do not see a physician for routine complaints. Once acclimated to this new system of care, most members of the prepaid group practice HMO seem to like it (as indicated by re-enrollment statistics), but the initial reaction is often negative.

An additional marketing problem for the new prepaid group practice HMO is the fact that it is a product without a local track record. Consumers are often hesitant to experiment with new products; when it comes to medical care, the response is intensified. For example, the Harvard Community Health Plan (case 2), despite the advantage of the Harvard name as an indicator of quality, had serious trouble initially with its marketing.

The performance of the well-established prepaid group practice HMOs has been good. Their hospital utilization rates are low compared to control groups, and their premiums are competitive.[10] One study has shown that they are creating competitive pricing pressures for traditional health insurers,[11] and bringing some change to their communities:

> There's some evidence that when HMOs get up to about 20 to 25 percent level of penetration in the health care marketplace that they begin to have a deterrent effect on the increase in medical care costs. Where successful HMOs have grown, they stimulate others to develop. This has been particularly true in the Boston area, where many of the panelists indicate that they started because the Harvard Community Health Plan started. We're grateful for that and pleased that we're able to stimulate some competition.
>
> Gordon Moore

There is one environmental factor which can contribute to a successful marketing effort: a large number of employed people without established physician relationships. These are the people for whom the prepaid group practice HMO is likely to have the greatest appeal, since the primary market for most HMOs is the employed population, and the prepaid group practice plan provides easy access to a complete medical system. Conversely, the prepaid group practice HMO will have a difficult marketing problem in an area where it must persuade a large number of people to break established ties with local physicians.

Companies contemplating sponsorship of a prepaid group practice HMO should be optimistic when one or more of the following conditions is present. The first is a shortage of physicians in the area, with residents experiencing difficulty locating physicians who will accept new patients. This was apparently the situation in Winston-Salem, North Carolina, when R. J. Reynolds founded its HMO.

The second condition is rapid growth in local population, particularly within the young adult age bracket. This has been the trend in California over the last several decades, and has probably contributed to the success of HMOs generally in that state.

A third condition which can be favorable is a rapid turnover in population, again particularly among young adults. This is a characteristic of Boston, with its large number of educational institutions and large proportion of professionals. The Harvard Community Health Plan has drawn heavily on these population groups for its membership.

Multispecialty Group Practice HMOs

A variation on the salaried group theme is the HMO which builds on one or more existing multispecialty group practices in a community. Each group contracts with the HMO to deliver all medical services to HMO members who choose the group as their source of care. The group receives payment on a

CASE 2

Harvard Community Health Plan

HMO Type: Salaried group (staff model)

Location: Greater Boston, Massachusetts

Original sponsor(s): University

Starting date: October 1969

Service area population: 2,500,000

Enrollment: 77,000

Participating physicians: 75 (Full-time equivalents)

In the late 1960s Harvard Medical School established a prepaid group practice plan in order to expand its service delivery programs, to test new approaches to the delivery and financing of medical care, and to provide a primary care training site. Incorporated as a free-standing, nonprofit entity, with a board of directors representing consumer groups, the public, Harvard University, and affiliated hospitals, the Harvard Community Health Plan was designed as a salaried group (staff model) HMO. Program development and initial operation were financed by loans of several hundred thousand dollars from Harvard Medical School and grants from the Commonwealth Fund, Rockefeller Foundation, and Ford Foundation, totaling $1.5 million. The first center was opened in Boston in the fall of 1969.

Until the passage of state HMO enabling legislation in 1976, HMO coverage in Massachusetss had to be issued by an insurance company. Since the plan did not have the capital reserves required to be an insurance company, it became affiliated with several carriers, primarily Blue Cross. Program directors also felt that working through the carriers would provide better access to the group insurance market and give the Plan some credibility in the eyes of potential purchasers. In addition to marketing, the carriers agreed to reinsure health care costs incurred by the plan in excess of 120 percent of the per-member projections and to provide administrative services (such as billing, premium collection, and claims processing).

The efforts of these insurers to enroll members prior to the program's inauguration were disappointing. Despite a mild penalty clause tied to enrollment quotas, enrollment levels remained so low after the center opened that the plan, with its high operating costs, faced the prospect of bankruptcy. This poor performance by the marketing agents was attributed in part to the mixed incentives of the insurers. They had no capital investment at risk, aggressive marketing might damage their relations with accounts, and enrollment in the plan was customarily achieved by cannibalizing existing group policy subscribers. Furthermore, the agents charged with marketing the plan had only a limited understanding of it.

The Harvard Community Health Plan thus found it necessary to overhaul its marketing approach within a few months of opening its doors. The contract with Blue Cross was modified to require the commitment of full-time staff to selling the plan, membership quotas were raised, and Blue Cross assumed responsibility for helping to meet fixed costs if enrollment quotas were not met. In addition, the plan hired its own marketing staff to approach non-Blue Cross accounts and to work cooperatively with the Blue Cross staff.

Training under the direction of plan management and medical staff was provided to both in-house and Blue Cross marketers. As a result of these measures, the marketing effort began to pay off, and sufficient enrollment was achieved to avert the closing of the plan. By the end of the third year of operation, approximately 30,000 individuals were enrolled. A second ambulatory facility was constructed, this one located in Boston's neighboring city of Cambridge, and enrollment has since continued to grow.

In 1977, with legal flexibility provided by a state HMO enabling act, the plan terminated its agreements with Blue Cross and the commercial insurers and switched to direct contracting with subscriber groups and in-house performance of services formerly provided by the insurance companies. Federal qualification was obtained in 1977, and plans are now being made to expand into the Boston suburbs with an application filed for authorization to construct a third ambulatory care facility. This expansion has been delayed by significant opposition by some local physicians to the granting of privileges to plan physicians at suburban hospitals.

Hospital utilization by plan members is approximately 350 days per 1,000; when adjusted for age and sex differences in comparison with the general population, plan utilization is still about 50 percent of the general rate. As a result, premiums for the plan are frequently lower than those for comprehensive traditional insurance plans. Similarly, the state reports cost savings of approximately 20 percent for Medicaid recipients enrolled in the Harvard Community Health Plan.

Sources

Robert S. Lurie and Robert L. Biblo, "HCHP Success and Failures in Communicating Information to Its Publics," in *Health Services and Health Hazards: The Employee's Need to Know*, Richard H. Egdahl and Diana Chapman Walsh, eds., Springer Series on Industry and Health Care, No. 4 (New York: Springer-Verlag, 1978), pp. 134–145.

Gordon Moore, Medical Director, Cambridge Health Center, Harvard Community Health Plans, and

Joel Abrams, Director of Community Health Services, Massachusetts Rate Setting Commission, Chairman, Massachusetts HMO Task Force, presentations at "Industry and HMOs in Massachusetts," a conference held by Boston University Center for Industry and Health Care, and Massachusetts Society of Internal Medicine, Boston, April 13, 1978.

Howard Waitzkin and Alana S. Cohen, "HMOs: A Critical Appraisal of The Harvard Community Health Plan." *Harvard Medical Alumni Bulletin* 47 (1972): 12–18.

Joseph L. Dorsey, "Commentary," *Harvard Medical Alumni Bulletin* **47** (1972): 19–21.

Ann S. Bush, *Group Practice: Planning and Implementing a Community-wide Prepayment Plan for Health Services*. New York, New York State Health Planning Commission, 1971, p. 27.

Roger W. Birnbaum, "The Harvard Community Health Plan: To Provide Broad Access to Quality, Comprehensive Care," *Public Welfare* 20:1 (January 1971): 42–46.

Joseph L. Dorsey, "Harvard Community Health Plan," *Massachusetts Physician* (May 1969): 36–38.

capitation basis for these HMO members. A multispecialty group practice HMO is similar to a prepaid group practice HMO, except in the degree to which they provide medical services on a fee-for-service basis to non-HMO members. The physicians in the group usually receive a salary, often adjusted based on productivity and the overall performance of the group. Thus, while the multispecialty group practice receives both capitation and fee-for-service income, payment to the physicians in the group is on a salaried basis. An example of a multispecialty group practice HMO is the Fallon Community Health Plan in Worcester, Massachusetts (case 3).

The basic advantage of the multispecialty group practice HMO is that it performs very much like a prepaid group practice, but without the need for a large investment in new facilities. Furthermore, the revenues from the existing fee-for-service business allow the group to maintain a larger number and variety of physicians without financial strain than is the case in the new salaried group HMO. This fee-for-service revenue also provides a cushion in case the group experiences some adversity in the early years of operation of the HMO, such as higher than expected utilization of services or low enrollment. A large group practice has a planning capacity:

The program at the Fallon Clinic is programmed to increase with our membership. Physicians are added as the population grows. We anticipated with reasonable assurance that we would need about one doctor per 1,000 covered population. So we keep the supply of physicians and ancillary personnel as close as we can to the actual need.

John O'Connell*

Another advantage of the multispecialty group practice HMO is that it avoids some of the marketing problems associated with new prepaid group practice HMOs. The group is already known to many consumers in the community. If the group's reputation is good, marketing is facilitated. In addition, the fact that a large number of people have used the group in the past minimizes the task of persuading others to join the new plan.

Industry involvement in multispecialty group practice HMO development has thus far been limited to support and encouragement, rather than direct sponsorship, as exemplified by the Twin City Health Care Development Project in Minneapolis, which became the National Association of Employers on Health Maintenance Organizations.[12] The Minneapolis project provided technical assistance to groups interested in joining HMOs, worked with the Minnesota legislature to pass HMO-enabling legislation, and provided marketing assistance to the HMOs which were subsequently developed.

Multispecialty groups are fairly widespread, with approximately 3,000 operating in the United States.[13] Of these, some 375 already receive prepayment revenue.[14] There should be considerable potential for the development of more HMOs among the remaining multispecialty groups.

Fee-for-Service HMOs

The fee-for-service HMO is the product of the physicians service bureaus, established in the Pacific Northwest in the early 1900s, and the foundations for medical care, founded in California in the mid-1950s. The former were essentially physician-sponsored health insurers, and the latter consisted of physician organizations emphasizing quality assurance through peer review.

The underlying goal of the fee-for-service HMO is to preserve certain aspects of the traditional medical care delivery system, while using prepayment with fixed dollars to control the cost of medical care. As in the traditional system, physicians serve as independent practitioners and continue to be paid on a fee-for-service basis. HMO members can choose from a large number of participating physicians—generally most, if not all, of the physicians in the area.

The fee-for-service HMO guarantees access to and delivery of comprehensive medical care services to members for a prepaid premium. The physician component guarantees delivery of medical services in return for a portion of the premium, and the physicians jointly assume the financial risk of providing those services. Moreover, they agree to participate in, and be bound

*Executive Director, Fallon Community Health Plan

CASE 3

Fallon Community Health Plan

HMO Type: Multispecialty group practice

Location: Worcester, Massachusetts (metropolitan area)

Original sponsor(s): Carrier and physicians

Starting date: February 1977

Service area population: 375,000

Enrollment: 6,000

Participating physicians: 40

The Fallon Clinic, founded in 1929, is a fee-for-service multispecialty group practice, representing about 10 percent of physicians in the Worcester area of Massachusetts. Beginning in 1973, representatives of the clinic met with Blue Cross of Massachusetts, which writes two-thirds of the group health insurance in the area, to discuss the possibility of establishing an HMO using the Fallon Clinic as its medical group, with underwriting and administrative support from Blue Cross. The Fallon Community Health Plan was incorporated as a nonprofit entity in 1975, with a six-member board of directors equally divided between clinic and Blue Cross representatives. Formal developmental work was accomplished with support from the federal HMO program.

Although not yet federally qualified, the plan became operational in February 1977. It purchases most health care services from the Clinic, which has a main outpatient facility in Worcester and a satellite facility to the east, in the Town of Westboro. The clinic receives a monthly capitation payment from the plan as compensation for all covered health care services except inpatient hospitalization, out-of-area emergency services, and certain subspecialties. Clinic physicians receive a salary, with incentive arrangements, from the clinic for both their HMO and non-HMO services. Inpatient hospital services are provided primarily at two hospitals which contract directly with the plan. Blue Cross pays all hospital claims and is reimbursed by the plan. If hospital utilization exceeds the budgeted level of 600 days per 1,000, the excess is paid by Blue Cross, under a reinsurance agreement with the plan. If hospital utilization is below 600 days per 1,000, the clinic receives a bonus payment from the plan. Current utilization is approximately 510 days of hospital care per 1,000 enrollees per year.

In addition to providing administrative and underwriting support for operation of the plan, Blue Cross staff provided an important source of technical assistance during the development phase. Under contract with the plan, Blue Cross receives capitation payments for its administrative and underwriting services. Although the plan employs its own marketing director, it contracts with Blue Cross for a designated minimum number of Blue Cross sales agents to work full time under the direction of the marketing director. Blue Cross also has agreed to enrollment quotas, or guarantees, for the plan. Additional Blue Cross services to the plan include premium billing and collection, individual stop-loss reinsurance, payment of out-of-area emergency and inpatient hospital claims, and provision of designated management reports. So it may meet operating deficits and provide adequate financial protection while awaiting qualification and eligibility for federal operating loans, Blue Cross has also extended a $250,000 line of credit to the plan.

During its first year and a half of operation, the plan enrolled 6,000 members. To insure that these enrollees receive high-quality health care, the Plan performs medical audits on samples of problem-oriented medical records, compares projected and actual treatment of designated conditions, and concurrently reviews each hospital admission on a daily basis. Audits of records are performed by a committee of clinic physicians, and hospital review is currently conducted by the plan's medical director. However, it is expected that a nurse will soon be employed to assume routine hospital review responsibilities, with physician support. Referrals to outside consultants are also recorded and reviewed periodically to monitor physician practices and assess the need for expanded in-house physician resources.

Sources

John P. O'Connell, Executive Director, Fallon Community Health Plan, personal communication, August 1978; presentation at "Industry and HMOs in Massachusetts," a conference held by Boston University Center for Industry and Health Care and Massachusetts Society of Internal Medicine, Boston, April 13, 1978.

by, peer review of their medical practices. Thus, the fee-for-service HMO provides physicians with a different set of incentives:

> Physicians, as the primary decision makers, have no incentives whatsoever to keep costs down under traditional insurance plans. In fact, almost everything they do involves incentives in the opposite direction. One of the most important strategies for cost control is to tie the physicians' incomes to the economic consequences of their decisions.
>
> Edmond Charrette*

> What the Bay State Health Care Foundation did is to say to the physicians, "If you want your prevailing rate, which we think you should have, the only way you are going to get it is if you can control costs."
>
> Gary Janko**

Fee-for-service HMOs can be grouped into four categories in a two-by-two matrix, according to the locus of control and the organizational structure. The HMO is controlled either by its participating physicians or by another party, such as an insurance carrier or a community board of directors. In terms of structure, either the physicians are members of a legally separate organization (like an IPA) which contracts with the HMO, or the physicians can contract directly with the HMO. Since the IPA model is the only type of fee-for-service HMO which qualifies under federal law, it is the predominant model. Similarly, since most fee-for-service HMOs are founded by organized medicine, they are usually controlled by the physicians.

A typical IPA type of fee-for-service HMO which is controlled by physicians is the Rocky Mountain HMO in Grand Junction, Colorado (case 4); Greater Delaware Valley Health Care, Inc. in Pennsylvania (case 5) is an IPA type controlled by a group other than the physicians. Examples of fee-for-service HMOs which contract directly with physicians are the Physicians Association of Clackamus County, sponsored by the county medical society,[15] and the North Central Health Protection Plan, sponsored by Employees Insurance of Wausau.[16]

The key to the success of a fee-for-service HMO is a combination of peer review and risk-sharing mechanisms designed to control the utilization and cost of providing medical services. For purposes of informal peer review, the HMO generally distributes monthly or other regular reports to participating physicians. Beyond detailing the financial status of the HMO, these reports often include a summary statement of the practice patterns of all the physicians, usually grouped by specialty, to allow them to compare their own performance to that of their peers. In some plans, the names of individual physicians are listed on the report, while in others random identifying numbers

---

*Immediate Past President, Massachusetts Society of Internal Medicine; Assistant Clinical Professor, Boston University School of Medicine.
**Executive Director, Bay State Health Care Foundation.

are used. The summary includes such information as average number of visits per patient, numbers of various diagnostic tests per visit, average cost per visit, and total cost per physician. The physicians study these reports carefully:

> One of the things the physicians look at, and spend probably 75 percent of their time on, is ambulatory care. They receive a physician's profile on a monthly basis that compares physicians in certain categories. This was their choice. We started out running a summary of all the physicians in the community, comparing them in certain categories by name, and sending it to all physicians. So every physician took a look at other members—at what they were doing, including such things as how many admissions, therapeutic injections, tests, x-rays they ordered. Gross exceptions not only stood out to the peer review committee, but also to every other physician in the community. And that's peer review! Practice habits change without anybody saying much of anything.
>
> Jacob J. Spies*

Formal peer review is performed by committees of participating physicians, which review in detail the practice decisions of physicians singled out for special attention. These might include physicians whose practice patterns appear to be out of line in summary reports, or those cited in specific complaints. The committees may also review a random sample of all cases and then follow up with more intensive reviews of those physicians identified as over-utilizers by that sample. Although the primary purpose of this peer review process is quality control, it also aids in controlling costs. Services identified as unnecessary either are not paid for or, if payment has already been made, are charged against future payments to the physician in question. Also, peer review provides a mechanism for modifying the behavior of participating physicians and encouraging cost consciousness. Finally, the peer review process identifies physicians who require sterner sanctions, such as suspension or termination. Several fee-for-service HMOs have used this sanction.

Peer review, both formal and informal, is essentially a retrospective process based on accumulated claims information. The fee-for-service HMO reviews claims as they are submitted, prior to payment. A minimal claims review system provides a check on administrative details, such as eligibility of the patient and whether the fee charged is within the allowable limits. More sophisticated systems also check on the appropriateness of the services provided for the diagnosis listed on the claim through comparison to predetermined treatment guidelines.

Claims which do not fall within the guidelines are reviewed by the medical director or other trained personnel, and payment is made only for approved services. Under the terms of the physician's contract with the IPA or HMO, the physician may not bill the patient for services which are not approved. The Bay State Health Care Foundation's proposal is an example of this kind of careful review of physician's claims:

---

* Vice President, Division of Health Care Systems, Employers Insurance of Wausau.

CASE 4

Rocky Mountain Health Maintenance Organization

HMO Type: Fee-for-service IPA

Location: Mesa County, Colorado

Original Sponsor(s): Physicians

Starting date: January 1974

Service area population: 66,000

Enrollment: 11,000

Participating physicians: 82

The Medical Society of Mesa County, Colorado began exploring HMO alternatives in 1971 for three specific reasons. First, the physicians wished to maintain and exercise local control over the way in which medicine was practiced in their community. Second, they wanted to deal collectively with the government bureaucracies handling the Medicare and Medicaid programs, and thus reduce the paperwork required of individual physicians. Third, they sought a better approach to the financing of health care for the non-Medicaid eligible poor. The initial study concluded that the development of a salaried group HMO was not feasible in Mesa County because of its rural character, the absence of existing group practices, and the high development and overhead costs that would be incurred. However, there was local and federal support for the development of a fee-for-service IPA-HMO. The program became operational in January 1974 with about 65 participating physicians and 3,400 enrollees (including 3,200 Medicaid recipients). Federal qualification was obtained after additional development work at the end of 1975.

In compliance with requirements for federal qualification, the IPA and the HMO are legally distinct organizations linked by contractual agreements. The IPA agrees to provide a medical director for the program and, through its participating physicians (82 of a total of 110 in Mesa County as of March 1978), to provide medical services to HMO enrollees, as well as professional review of the medical care delivered. Each enrollee selects a primary care physician who makes referrals for any required specialty care.

Business aspects of the program, such as marketing, financial monitoring, premium collection, and compliance with federal reporting requirements, are the responsibility of the HMO. The all-physician board of directors of the IPA holds a majority of the seats on the HMO's board, giving the participating physicians a strong voice in all aspects of program operations.

The HMO compensates the IPA, which in turn pays the physicians, on a fee-for-service basis according to a fee schedule, with 10 percent (formerly 20 percent) of fees withheld by the HMO for deposit in a risk account used to cover unbudgeted expenses (medical, hospital, administrative, and so on) or to build reserves. If unneeded for either of these purposes, the risk account is distributed to the participating physicians. Unlike some other plans, however, if the HMO has a surplus in its hospital fund at year's end, the physicians do not share in it.

The program was originally designed to control hospital utilization through a combination of incentives (the doctors could lose the 20 percent of their fees withheld if hospital costs were higher than budgeted) and concurrent and retrospective utilization review. Despite promising first-year results, however, hospital utilization climbed during the first half of 1975. Analysis revealed that although the concurrent review program was holding down the average length of stay of hospitalized enrollees, the admission rate was unacceptably high. To combat this problem, a mandatory hospital preadmission certification program for all elective cases was instituted in mid-1975. The rate of hospital utilization dropped rapidly, as a result, and utilization in 1977 was approximately 560 days per 1,000 compared to about 800 days per 1,000 during early 1975.

In just over four years, the program has expanded its market share from 6 to 17 percent of the 66,000 residents of Mesa County, including 8,000 who are not Medicaid enrollees. In October 1977, Rocky Mountain HMO began to break even financially and has operated "in the black" since. As one outcome of this improved financial picture, the HMO is preparing to distribute part of its accumulated reserves to the participating physicians.

Sources

Michael Weber, Executive Director, Rocky Mountain Health Maintenance Organization, personal communication, March and August 1978.

Michael Weber, "Rocky Mountain HMO," in National Conference on Individual Practice Associations (Stockton, California: American Association of Foundations for Medical Care, 1977), pp. 79–88.

Harry L. Sutton, Jr., George V. Stennes and Associates, Minneapolis, Minnesota, testimony at hearing on Bay State Health Care Foundation held by Massachusetts Division of Insurance, Boston, May 12, 1978.

Member's Handbook (Grand Junction, Colorado: Rocky Mountain Health Maintenance Organization, August 1977).

CASE 5

Greater Delaware Valley Health Care, Inc.

HMO Type: Fee-for-service IPA

Location: Delaware County and vicinity, Pennsylvania

Original Sponsor(s): Corporate

Starting date: April 1978

Service area population: 620,000

Enrollment: 1,600

Participating physicians: 300

In the early 1970s the Sun Company, a major employer in Delaware County, southwest of Philadelphia, began to search for strategies that would help control its rising health care expenditures. Several closed-panel group practice plans were located in Philadelphia, but with their limited accessibility, they were not judged to be attractive to the work force. In order to catalyze the development of an HMO in Delaware County, the Sun Company first approached the largest local hospital, then contacted other large employers and hospitals. As a result, twenty-four companies expressed interest in cooperating in a study to determine if the existing health care resources serving Delaware County could be rearranged to form an HMO. A committee consisting of employer, provider, union, and community representatives was formed to oversee the study.

During the course of the feasibility study, which was funded by nine companies, it soon became evident that there was practically no multispecialty group activity in the county, and that the physicians had no interest in forming such practices. However, physicians on the staffs of several hospitals indicated an interest in forming individual practice associations, and in a number of instances this was paralleled by hospital interest in an HMO. According to information provided by the employers, a sufficient local market existed, in terms of numbers of employees and health insurance coverage, to support an HMO.

Although the feasibility study was completed by the end of 1974, the development phase was prolonged by difficulties of raising funds, first from the private sponsors and then through federal grants, opposition by some local physicians, and the complexity of the program structure. It was not until April 1978 that Greater Delaware Valley Health Care, Inc. commenced operations. An application for federal qualification is pending.

Greater Delaware Valley Health Care, Inc. uses three distinct IPAs, each composed of the members of the medical staff of one of three participating hospitals (staff participation rates vary between 50 and 90 percent). Each enrollee selects a primary care physician, who is affiliated with a particular IPA-hospital pair. For each IPA-hospital pair, the HMO sets up a physician fund and a hospital fund, both on a capitation formula. While the capitation rate for the three physician funds is the same, a different rate is used for each of the three hospital funds. Hospital capitation rates are determined by a formula that takes into account each hospital's costs (as reflected by the facility's Blue Cross rate), as well as a uniform budgeted utilization rate (600 days per 1,000 enrollees).

Under the terms of the compensation arrangements, both the participating physicians and the hospital in each IPA-hospital pair accept financial risk. Physicians are paid for their services on a fee-for-service basis according to a common fee schedule from the physician fund of the IPA to which the patient's primary physician belongs. Fifteen percent of the negotiated fees are withheld for deposit in a risk account to protect against unbudgeted physician expenses.

Each hospital draws on a per diem basis from the hospital fund of the participating facility with which the patient's primary physician's IPA is paired. Hospitals are obligated to return to the HMO any payment received in excess of their prevailing charges as part of a year-end settlement. Year-end surpluses in each facility's hospital fund must first be used to meet any deficit in the physician fund of the associated IPA. Additional surpluses are shared by the IPA (25 percent), the hospital (50 percent), and the HMO (25 percent). Surpluses in the physician fund must be used to offset any deficit of the associated hospital, with the remainder, if any, retained by the IPA. If these surplus dollars are insufficient to offset the total deficit in the hospital fund, any monies remaining in the risk account, after physicians have been compensated up to a minimum of 95 percent of the fee schedule, are used to meet the remaining deficit.

Greater Delaware Valley Health Care, Inc. is an independent, nonprofit, health plan. Its board of directors includes members chosen by employers offering the HMO, unions representing employees at companies offering the HMO, subscribers, and participating physicians and hospitals. It is anticipated that the plan will break even when it reaches an enrollment of approximately 14,000, projected for 1982 or 1983.

Sources

John Nelson, Executive Director, Greater Delaware Valley Health Care, Inc., personal communication, May and August 1978.

"How Business Helped in Delaware Valley to Set Up an Innovative Health Plan Despite Some Opposition," Health Cost Containment (May 14, 1978): 1–2.

Charles S. Ryan, Corporate Medical Director, Sun Company, Inc., presentation at "The Secretary's National HMO Conference," sponsored by the U.S. Department of Health, Education, and Welfare in Washington, D.C., March 10, 1978.

Plan materials: Member Handbook, "Backgrounder," "Legal History and Current Legal Status," "Hospital Services Agreement," "Medical Services Agreement," and "The Health Plan" (Radnor, Pennsylvania: Greater Delaware Valley Health Care, Inc.).

We've developed a 1,500-page set of medical care guide-lines which in fact are used by other IPA programs. It covers 80 percent of the medical diagnoses that would appear throughout the population, and allows us to do very stringent peer reviews. We've developed a management information system that allows us to control for the fact that initially a small percentage of the physicians' patient population will be members of the Bay State Health Care Plan. We reduce everything to a cost per service per patient by diagnosis. After all of that management information is accumulated and displayed, and we've had a chance to review the necessity of the claims for services, then the physician gets paid. If we decide, or the physician's peers decide, that the services rendered were not necessary, the claim doesn't get paid, and the patient doesn't get billed. The doctor has no choice but to look at his own practice pattern.

Gary Janko

Many fee-for-service HMOs intervene to prevent the performance of unnecessary services and avoid incurring the associated costs. The primary focus of such mechanisms is hospitalization, which must be controlled if the HMO is to survive. There are programs designed to control the two components of total days of hospitalization: admissions and length of stay. (Hospital days per 1,000 members per year is the product of admissions per 1,000 members per year times average length of stay per admission.) The surest way to control admissions is through a preadmission certification program, which requires that the physician obtain the permission of the HMO prior to putting any HMO member in the hospital, except in the case of an emergency. Since preadmission certification programs represent a major change in the way physicians practice, they are often not used in fee-for-service HMOs. However, plans which have had major problems with overutilization, such as Physicians Health Plan of Greater Minneapolis (case 6), have usually instituted preadmission certification as part of their recovery program.

Length of stay is controlled by a concurrent review program, in which each patient is assigned an expected length of stay based on the average length of stay for that diagnosis in the geographic area. The physician who wishes to keep a patient in the hospital for a longer period must apply to the utilization review committee of either the hospital or the HMO, depending on the locus of the program, for an extension. Usually, a short extension is routinely granted, but a second request is thoroughly reviewed. Preadmission certification programs and concurrent review programs are often used in tandem, with the preadmission program automatically assigning an expected length of stay which is used in the concurrent review program.

These two programs are accompanied by a set of sanctions for the physician and the patient, depending on the HMO and the circumstances. Generally, physicians will not be paid for any services they may render in violation of the program. If the physician has failed to follow the procedures, the patient is not held responsible, and the HMO pays the hospital bill. In some plans, the physician fund is responsible for payment of hospital bills involving violation of procedures, and in some cases the physician must pay such bills. The patient is liable if admission is denied under the preadmission certification program, and the patient and physician decide to proceed with hospitalization. If the patient wishes to remain in the hospital after being informed under the concurrent review program that the stay will no longer be covered, then the patient is responsible for the portion of the bill covering extended hospitalization.

Finally, the HMO exercises some control over the use of certain ambulatory services, such as referrals to specialists, hospital outpatient departments, and emergency rooms. An increasingly popular method is to use a "lock-in" to primary care physicians. At the time of enrollment, the new HMO member chooses a participating primary care physician to act as the "manager" of the member's medical care. The physician agrees to provide, or arrange for the provision of, all medical care services required by that member, and the member agrees not to seek any medical services not provided for or arranged by the primary physician, except for emergency services. The lock-in method is analogous to the relationship between a salaried group and its subscribers. Of course, the member has the option of changing primary physicians, with proper notification to the HMO, and is then locked in with the new participating physician.

The lock-in is designed both to give the member the same kind of coordinated, continuous care provided by a salaried group HMO and to give the HMO some management control over use of medical services. The primary care physician can make appropriate decisions on the need for referral physicians, and can make an informed judgment as to which of the available specialists is the best choice for the particular case. The lock-in discourages the member from shopping for care at several sites, such as specialists' offices, hospital outpatient departments, and emergency rooms. Some plans require prior ap-

CASE 6

Physicans Health Plan

HMO Type: Fee-for-service

Location: Greater Minneapolis, Minnesota

Original sponsor(s): Physicians

Starting date: August 1975

Service area population: 1,930,000

Enrollment: 25,000

Participating physicians: 1,200

By the end of 1974, the greater Minneapolis area had become a center of HMO activity, with six salaried group HMOs, of which five had commenced operations during the previous three years. During this period, enrollment had doubled in these plans, to a total of 84,000 members, and community acceptance was growing rapidly. Assessing the long-term threat of the group plans to their practices, the physicians in private practice decided that their best strategy would be to establish a competitive fee-for-service HMO. Under the sponsorship of the Hennepin County Medical Society, the Physicians Health Plan was incorporated in December 1974. By August 1975, when the first services were provided, approximately 1,200 physicians within a six-county area had signed contracts with the HMO.

As originally structured, the program assumed that the financial incentive to the physicians of having 20 percent of their fees held at risk to meet any losses incurred would be sufficient to effect a voluntary shift in physician behavior toward greater cost consciousness and control. However, because physicians had been recruited on the premise that the plan would enable them to continue to practice in their customary style, and in the absence of a formal utilization review and control system, this assumption proved unrealistic. By March 1976, the plan's physician-dominated board of directors was informed by the staff of serious financial problems; however, because of the perception that the claims experience available was too preliminary and limited, no action was taken. Within the next eight months, during which time enrollment increased rapidly, the plan's cash needs became acute and remedial action could no longer be postponed. In order to meet nonphysician claims, loans had to be obtained from a local insurance company and, by the end of 1976, the proportion of physicians' fees withheld had been increased to 30 percent.

Excessive hospital utilization was the most important factor contributing to the plan's financial problems. To reduce utilization, a program was instituted requiring prospective certification of hospital admissions and justification of the length of stay. There were, however, no sanctions for noncompliance, so participating physicians seldom requested the plan's approval before hospitalizing patients. By mid-1977 the plan had incurred a deficit of over a half million dollars, and the management firm hired to administer the plan informed the board of directors that controls would have to be tightened and supported by penalties if the organization was to remain solvent. With little real alternative if the plan was to remain a competitive force, the board instituted tight utilization review policies.

Now, participating physicians are denied payment if they fail to obtain prior authorization from the plan either for non-emergency hospital admissions, or for extending a hospital stay beyond the initially certified number of days. A full-time nurse coordinator has been employed to implement the utilization review system and to monitor compliance. Severe restrictions have also been placed on referrals to nonparticipating physicians, and the plan has entered into a contractual arrangement with a local clinic to provide, or arrange for, the rich benefits for mental health care and chemical dependency services required under Minnesota law. Additionally, the ambulatory care practice patterns (such as visits per patient, and cost per visit) of individual plan physicians are now compared to those of other participating physicians in the same specialty. Physicians exceeding the plan's norms by a certain amount are required to refund the excess revenues to the plan; otherwise, they are dropped from the plan.

Although these controls have placed a strain on the plan's relationship with some of its participating physicians (about 1 percent of whom resigned from the plan when the controls were implemeted), almost all have made the necessary adjustments. One contributing factor to this acceptance is undoubtedly the continued success of the salaried group HMOs in the area, which have attracted 100,000 additional members since the end of 1974. The controls have also been effective. Annualized inpatient hospital utilization, which averaged approximately 750 days per 1,000 enrollees in 1977, has been reduced to under 650 days per 1,000 in 1978. Moreover, the plan reports that it has operated "in the black" in every month since the more stringent controls and sanctions were implemented, that the accumulated deficit from development and operations has been all but eliminated, and that the portion of physicians' fees withheld has been returned to 20 percent. Obtaining better control of costs has also enabled the plan to maintain competitive premium rates, and enrollment has grown from 10,000 at the beginning of 1977 to 25,000 in July, 1978.

Sources

Richard T. Burke, Executive Director, Physicians Health Plan, testimony at hearing on Bay State Health Care Foundation held by Massachusetts Division of Insurance, Boston, May 12, 1978; and personal communication, August 1978.

Karen Hunt, "The Painful Truth About Prepayment," *American Medical News, Impact* (June 23, 1978): 6–7.

Steven B. Enright, "Beating HMOs At Their Own Game," *Medical Economics* (June 10, 1978): 97–111.

"Tight Controls on IPA Physicians Turn Around Plan's Deficit Troubles," *Health Services Information* V:2 (January 16, 1978): 2–3.

Jon B. Christianson, *The Competitive Impact of Health Maintenance Organizations: Minneapolis-St. Paul* (Excelsior, Minnesota: InterStudy, undated).

proval for specialist referrals, particularly those to nonparticipating specialists or to hospital clinics. Some plans also require large co-payments for inappropriate use of the emergency room.

The physicians in a fee-for-service HMO are at financial risk for the services to HMO members, both on an individual and group basis. Every physician is at risk for his own services, since payment will not be made if the HMO finds such services unnecessary. The individual physician is also at risk for the performance of all other participating physicians, because a percentage of all physician billings to the HMO is withheld to create a reserve account. The portion withheld is generally between 10 and 20 percent; it may be changed by vote of the board of directors of the IPA or HMO. Some plans, such as Mastercare in Albuquerque, have had to withhold 30 percent or more to meet unexpected financial needs of the HMO.[17]

The reserve created in this manner covers greater-than-budgeted use of physician services, primarily paying for overutilization of physician services and any other services which are the responsibility of the physicians. Also, the reserve often covers a portion of the overutilization of services paid for by other components of the HMO, such as hospitalization. After all expenses are covered, the balance of the risk fund at year's end may be distributed to the participating physicians on a pro-rata basis. Thus, if the HMO operates within its budgeted utilization of services, physicians will receive 100 percent of fees after the distribution. If overutilization occurs, then physicians will loose a portion of their billings. This risk-sharing arrangement acts as a reinforcing device for the peer review process. Since risk sharing creates joint responsibility for the financial results of individual medical decisions, the physicians have an incentive to conduct rigorous peer review.

If utilization is less than budgeted, the surplus is usually used to build reserves or to lower premiums and thereby improve the competitive position of te HMO in the marketplace. A surplus is generally not distributed to the participating physicians, since it would allow them to collect in excess of 100 percent of fees. Even HMOs or IPAs organized as for-profit organizations usually do not distribute the surplus, recognizing that it might provide a stimulus to physicians not to deliver necessary health care:

> In every year except 1974 there's been a surplus of 2 to 3 percent on the withhold for physicians' fees. In all seven plans, the interesting thing is that except for the first year, the physicians have not taken that surplus. They have always indicated that it had not been their intention to come out ahead on this thing.
>
> Jacob J. Spies

At the heart of virtually all of these programs is a management information system. The system used by the average fee-for-service HMO must keep track of the activities of all its members and physicians, as well as organize the raw claims and membership data to produce the various reports and other information required to operate the control programs. As a result, fee-for-service HMOs have made rapid progress in developing sophisticated computer software for their management information systems.

The fee-for-service HMO has several advantages for a company pursuing HMO development. First, it is the most acceptable form of HMO to the majority of practicing physicians. It provides the physicians an opportunity to continue practicing fee-for-service medicine, while removing some of the inappropriate incentives which are part of the traditional insurance programs. For example, the physician participating in a fee-for-service HMO no longer needs to hospitalize a patient for a diagnostic work-up, whereas traditionally hospitalization was required for coverage by an indemnity insurance plan. The fee-for-service HMO also simplifies administration through the use of precoded encounter forms, rather than the more cumbersome claim forms required by health insurers. Moreover, this type of HMO provides prompt payment, thus easing cash flow problems. Finally, there is no problem of bad debt for members.

Second, fee-for-service HMOs can be developed in most communities. Although it is easier to persuade physicians to accept the controls inherent in this type of HMO when there is a competitive threat from a salaried group HMO, the experience of the Employers Insurance of Wausau and the Rocky Mountain HMO indicates that this is not a necessary precondition. Furthermore, becasue the overhead costs of a fee-for-service HMO are lower than those of the salaried group type, the former can break even with a smaller membership. Break-even populations for fee-for-service HMOs range from 5,000 to 20,000 members; thus these plans are feasible in areas with populations which appear to be too small to support salaried group HMOs.

A third advantage of the fee-for-service HMO is its acceptability to a wide range of people. If the majority of physicians in an area participate, then most potential members will not have to change physicians to join the plan. Thus, the fee-for-service HMO can draw on a different, and often larger, market segment than the salaried group HMO. This segment is comprised of people with established relationships with physicians, and usually includes a large proportion of families and somewhat older adults. Since this same segment of the market is likely to represent a large proportion of the employed population, it is important to provide an HMO which will appeal to them.

An initial problem faced by the company interested in developing a fee-for-service HMO is how to approach area physicians. One strategy is to work with the local medical society or medical foundation. The advantages of this approach are access to an organized physician group and the immediate credibility of the new HMO afforded by its link with the medical society. In areas where the medical society has considerable influence, it may not be feasible to start an IPA if the medical society is lukewarm or opposed. The society will control at least the physician component and it may wish to control the HMO as well.

The problem with medical society control is that initially the society may be less likely to exercise rigorous utilization control than an organization formed specifically for that purpose. The medical society tends to be reluctant to impose sanctions on physicians who practice inefficient, but not low-quality, medicine, given organized medicine's traditional support of individuality in practice patterns. Some fee-for-service HMOs sponsored by medical societies, such as the Physicians Health Plan of Greater Minneapolis, have resisted imposing sanctions until forced by severe financial problems to instigate control measures. A medical society tie may also pose antitrust problems, since any fee schedule used by such a fee-for-service HMO could be considered a price-fixing tool, in the same manner as the relative value schedules which are now under attack by the Federal Trade Commission.[18] These are some of the issues that were raised in the Bay State Health Care Foundation hearings (appendix II).

Gary Janko believes the Bay State's regulatory problems are tied up with the dispute between Blue Shield of Massachusetts and the Massachusetts Medical Society over physician fees and contracts:

> A lot of the regulators say, "Gee, these greedy doctors—they want to form this IPA and get higher fees and get out from under Blue Shield." But that is not the reason physicians joined the program. They see it as a necessary, competitive force that's going to improve the health care of anybody who decides to enroll in it. That's the purpose.

A second strategy for approaching area physicians—used by the industry sponsors of the Greater Delaware Valley Health Care, Inc.—is to work with hospital medical staffs. Like the medical society, a hospital staff offers the advantage of a pre-existing medical organization; the likely model is the IPA. In a metropolitan area with many hospitals and physicians, the alliance may provide a means of organizing enough physicians to serve the HMO population by working with only a few of the available hospitals, thus avoiding development of a large, unwieldy organization, with all its inherent administrative problems. Further, if each hospital medical staff is organized as a separate IPA contracting with the HMO, then each IPA will constitute a reasonable peer group for the participating physicians. The question of the need for such smaller scale peer groups has been raised for very large fee-for-service HMOs, such as the Bay State Health Care Foundation. Working with hospital medical staffs necessarily involves bringing the hospitals into the HMO development process from the start, probably as partners. (The issue of hospital partnership is discussed later in this chapter.) Hospitals may be reluctant to help create HMOs, which are, after all, designed to reduce hospitalization. However, hospitals may also benefit from such development, either through increasing the population base that they serve or by sharing in the subsequent savings generated by fee-for-service HMOs, as discussed in chapter 5.

A third strategy is to identify a few leading physicians in the community and work with them to create a fee-for-service HMO as a new organization. This approach was used by Employers Insurance of Wausau. While forming a fee-for-service HMO in this manner may be a slower process than collaborating with a hospital staff or medical society, it may pay off in better physician understanding of, and commitment to, the fee-for-service HMO concept. The danger of working with pre-existing medical organizations is that physicians may be enrolled to participate simply as a result of their membership in the organization, and without a full understanding of their obligations in the fee-for-service HMO. The degree of physician commitment to the plan is critical, particularly if the HMO runs into problems in the first couple of years and has to make adjustments by tightening controls or increasing the risk reserve fund (that is, raising the percentage of fees withheld).

The above three strategies are not mutually exclusive, in the sense that industry will always look for physician leadership to help in the development process, whether that leadership is to be found in the medical society, the hospital medical staff, or respected community physicians. Similarly, in a one-hospital town, working through the medical society and working through the hospital medical staff may be synonymous. The point is that a company attempting to develop a fee-for-service HMO must analyze its environment and the medical community it will be working with to determine the best approach.

The fee-for-service HMO would seem to have greater potential for rapid growth than the salaried group HMO, since the former is less disruptive of present patterns of medical care delivery. The fee-for-service HMO provides the physician with a means of competing against the group practice HMOs without having to change his entire mode of practice. It offers the patient a system which can control costs without requiring a radical change in the traditional method of delivering medical care—a method which surveys show the patient generally finds satisfactory. Thus, the fee-for-service HMO should be readily acceptable to a community. And since it should be possible to organize this type of HMO in many more places than is the case for the group practice type, fee-for-service HMOs can be expected to develop in many areas.

Why, then, are there not many more fee-for-service HMOs serving large numbers of people? One reason is that the fee-for-service HMO is still a new idea, and it depends on physicians voluntarily tightening up their practice patterns—and taking cost into account more than has been necessary in the past. Most have been developed within the last five years and have not had a chance to prove themselves to physicians and consumers in the way that the Kaiser Foundation Health Plans have done over the last thirty years.

Also, many proponents of the salaried group HMOs, particularly those in organized labor, have been reluctant to endorse the idea of fee-for-service HMOs. The latter are often considered by the supporters of the group practice type as too conservative because of their reliance on fee-for-service payment. At the other extreme, organized medicine considers fee-for-service HMOs too radical in their stringent control of medical practice. Fortunately, these attitudes are changing as both sides begin to see the role that the fee-for-service HMO can play in bringing mainstream physicians into organizations designed to control costs.

Finally, there is often no organizing force for physicians, particularly in areas where there are no competing salaried group HMOs.

Other Emerging HMO Models

This last category includes the few plans which pay their physicians directly on a per-capita basis. These HMOs contract with primary care physicians (general practitioners, family practitioners, internists, pediatricians, and, sometimes, obstetricians/gynecologists) in the community to serve as the physician component. Each primary care physician is paid a capitation, often adjusted according to the patient's age and sex, for each HMO member who chooses the physician for primary care. The HMO member is then locked into a relationship with that primary care physician, in the same way that members of some fee-for-service HMOs are locked in. Also like the fee-for-service type, these plans rely on the physicians already practicing in a community and contract with a sufficiently dispersed number of physicians to assure widespread service. As with salaried group HMOs, physicians' incomes are unrelated to the volume of services they provide to members of the HMO.

The primary care physician is responsible for arranging for the services of specialists and for hospitalization for HMO members under his care. The physician's capitation pays for services of physicians to whom the member is referred, and covers most nonhospital services provided or ordered directly by the primary physician. Administratively, this is usually accomplished by the HMO retaining some portion of the capitation in a reserve account to cover the costs of referrals, which the HMO pays on a fee-for-service basis, and other services, such as laboratory and x-ray tests, covered in the physician's contract. At the end of the accounting period, which is usually annual, the surplus in this account is paid to the primary care physicians. Conversely, the physicians may be held responsible for covering deficits.

Several mechanisms are available to help minimize some of the financial risks of capitation for the primary care physician. For example, Northwest Healthcare in Seattle, sponsored by SAFECO Life Insurance Co., specifies that a physician must have at least fifty HMO members as patients to be eligible to participate in full capitation arrangements.[19] Setting such a minimum number reduces the risk for participating physicians. For a similar reason, the Group Health Plan of Northeast Ohio (case 7) prefers to deal with primary care groups, which accept members jointly, although it also contracts with individual physicians in certain instances. Some HMOs provide a phase-in period for the newly participating physician, wherein the risk is reduced, usually by means of a year-end adjustment limiting losses (and gains). The HMO may reinsure some of this physician's risk by providing individual stop-loss or aggregate loss coverage. These kinds of coverage can be offered directly by the HMO or through a reinsurance contract purchased in the commercial insurance market.

In addition, the physician sometimes bears part of the risk of greater-than-budgeted use of hospitalization, as in the Health Maintenance Organization of Pennsylvania (case 8). This control is useful because, otherwise, the physician could maximize his own return by hospitalizing patients. This incentive to hospitalize unnecessarily is removed by having the primary physician and the HMO share in the surpluses and deficits in the hospitalization account.

Often, the HMO does not directly control referrals, since it relies on the primary care physician to choose wisely with respect to price and quality. To insure that a bill received from a specialist or hospital actually represents an authorized service, the HMO uses some control mechanism. For example, the Group Health Plan of Northeast Ohio makes the primary care physician responsible for paying for all services which he authorizes. In general, the member must pay for any nonemergency care received without authorization from the primary care physician.

HMOs in this third category have both advantages and disadvantages. The direct capitation payment system clearly links physician behavior with economic rewards, since participating physicians do not jointly assume the risk of providing services within the budget, as they do in other HMOs. Simply in terms of financial incentives, physicians in the direct capitation type of HMO can be expected to minimize the cost of providing their patients with medical care. Thus, they would be expected to treat directly as many complaints as possible, rather than referring their patients to expensive specialists, and to order only those laboratory tests that are likely to provide useful information.

On the other hand, HMOs using direct capitation rely more heavily on each participating physician's professional judgment than on peer review programs. If carried to an extreme, the financial incentives built into the direct capitation system could result in poor quality of health care. For example, the primary care physician might treat patients with conditions outside his area of expertise, in order to avoid referrals, or might skimp on diagnostic testing. Balancing the incentives is important for all HMOs:

> I can see an incentive to do a little gynecology and a little ortho-
> pedics, maybe even try a little minor surgery, but one of the mech-
> anisms that I think serves as an effective barrier against too much

CASE 7

Group Health Plan of Northeast Ohio

HMO Type: Direct capitation

Location: Cleveland, Akron, Lorain and vicinity, Ohio

Original sponsor(s): Consumer and government

Starting date: April 1975

Service area population: 3,200,000

Enrollment: 11,000

Participating physicians: 55

The Group Health Plan of Northeast Ohio evolved from the Cleveland Community Health Network, an alternative health care delivery system supported by the Office of Economic Opportunity. Group Health Plan serves both publicly and privately financed populations through a network of primary care physicians in the Greater Cleveland-Akron-Lorain area. The HMO contracts with sixteen groups of from one to eight family practice or general practice physicians, some of which are components of larger multispecialty group practices. The HMO meets annually with the medical directors of all participating physician groups to negotiate a single capitation rate for all enrollees which will be acceptable to all the groups and to the HMO. The contract with each group specifies that this capitation payment is to be payment in full for all out-of-hospital and in-hospital physician services, including specialty care, as well as ambulatory and hospital outpatient laboratory work and x-rays.

Each family enrolling in the program chooses a participating general practice or family practice physician to serve as family physician. The medical group with which that physician is associated receives the capitation payments from the HMO for that family. If the family physician refers an HMO patient to a specialist, the medical group must pay any billing that results. Charges for other services covered by the capitation payment are also the responsibility of the medical group. Each medical group determines whether its primary physicians will be compensated for their HMO services on a fee-for-service or capitation basis.

Premium dollars remaining after the HMO has paid medical group capitations and administrative expenses, are retained by Group Health Plan to pay for all other services, such as skilled nursing facilities, home care, and inpatient hospital services. A separate hospital budget is established for each medical group. Hospital admission and length of stay are reviewed only retrospectively, and hospital utilization is controlled primarily by means of locking in the enrollee to the medical group. In addition, the HMO pays the medical group a bonus of 50 percent of any year-end surplus in the medical group's hospital budget, thereby providing an incentive for the group to exercise restraint in arranging or authorizing hospitalization. Currently, Group Health Plan of Northeast Ohio budgets for about 470 inpatient days per 1,000 enrollees annually, and actual utilization in 1977 was approximately 440 days per 1,000. A medical group is not responsible for making up any portion of a deficit in its hospital budget. Instead, the HMO purchases reinsurance, and maintains reserves and deposits with the state department of insurance to cover any hospital claims in excess of budget.

The program has had difficulty selling the capitation concept to the physicians, and some of the physicians (especially those located in the inner cities) believe that they are making less money under the capitation arrangement than they would be making on a fee-for-service basis. Nevertheless, the program has been sufficiently successful that other medical groups are now taking the initiative in making inquiries about participation under the plan.

Sources

Maxwell H. Davis, Executive Director, Group Health Plan of Northeast Ohio; and Dee Mc Pherran, Executive Secretary, Group Health Plan of Northeast Ohio, personal communication, April and August 1978.

Arthur Owens, "An HMO Setup Where Doctors Pay Doctors," *Medical Economics* (March 6, 1978): 131–137.

Plan materials: *Handbook for Members of Group Health Plan* and "Information About GHP" (Cleveland, Ohio: Group Health Plan of Northeast Ohio).

CASE 8

Health Maintenance Organization of Pennsylvania

HMO Type: Direct capitation

Location: Montgomery, Philadelphia, Bucks, Delaware, and Chester counties, Pennsylvania

Original sponsor(s): Consumer

Starting date: April 1977

Service area population: 3,800,000

Enrollment: 14,000

Participating physicians: 110 (IPA only)

In 1975 a consumer-sponsored organization was funded under the grant provisions of the federal HMO Act to develop a pre-paid system of health care delivery that would adapt existing resources to meet the needs of the residents of Philadelphia and four neighboring Pennsylvania counties. The sponsors, with support and input from local physician leaders, developed an IPA-HMO structure using direct capitation to participating primary care providers. Enrollees choose a primary care physician from participating family practitioners, internists, and pediatricians (obstetrician-gynecologists are not classified as primary physicians in this plan). These primary care physicians constitute the membership of the IPA, and they practice in their own offices which are dispersed throughout the HMO service area. Single-specialty groups of two to five physicians are most common, but solo practices are also represented.

The HMO collects premiums and pays a per capita amount to the IPA for all physician services. The IPA, in turn, makes a monthly capitation payment to each primary care physician for each HMO member under his or her care. The capitation payment, which varies with the member's age, covers all inpatient and outpatient primary care services. The balance of the funds received by the IPA are used to pay for specialists and to maintain a risk reserve fund. Specialist physicians sign service agreements with the IPA but are not members and are not at risk. Specialist physicians agree to provide services to enrollees when referred by the primary physician, and to accept payment on a fee-for-service basis from the IPA, according to a set fee schedule. Specialists' bills have the first claim on the risk reserve fund, should there be overutilization. Approximately 600 specialists have signed participation agreements.

The HMO also establishes accounts for paying other expenses, including hospitals, out-of-area coverage, and administrative costs. Hospital services are provided through per diem arrangements with approximately twenty area hospitals. The HMO has established a hospital utilization target of 520 days per 1,000 enrollees. If utilization exceeds this target, the balance of the IPA's risk reserve fund is used to offset 50 percent of excess hospital expenses. If hospital utilization is below target, a percentage of the savings is added to the risk reserve fund. After these adjustments are made, the IPA decides how to distribute the surplus, if any, to IPA member physicians.

Any physician may be excluded from sharing in the distribution of this fund if the IPA's medical review committee concludes that his practice pattern has directly or indirectly (through the decisions of referral physicians) exceeded IPA-established criteria without sufficient medical justification. The HMO staff, with the active encouragement and cooperation of the IPA, makes a substantial effort to assure that only those primary physicians who understand and agree with both the objectives of the program and the responsibilities of IPA membership, and whose styles of practice reflect this understanding and agreement, are accepted as IPA members. Some 25 percent of primary physicians who apply for IPA membership are rejected.

The Health Maintenance Organization of Pennsylvania has developed rapidly. It opened to members just twenty-one months after receiving its feasibility grant in July 1975, and became federally qualified less than three months later. Over 10,000 people were enrolled during the first year of operation. Annualized hospital utilization during the first quarter of 1978 was approximately 460 days per 1,000 enrollees.

Sources

Leonard Abramson, President, The Health Maintenance Organization of Pennsylvania, personal communication, May 1978, August 1978.

Michelle Kindt, Director of Quality Assurance, The Health Maintenance Organization of Pennsylvania, personal communication, May 1978.

Plan Materials: *Member Handbook,* "Primary Physician Agreement," "Specialist Physician Agreement," "The HMO of Pennsylvania Map," "Brief Summary," and letter from Associate Medical Director accompanying applications for IPA membership (Willow Grove, Pennsylvania: Health Maintenance Organization of Pennsylvania).

financial temptation to do things that the family practitioner is not capable of doing, is that the front line of specialists—obstetricians, gynecologists, general surgeons—really function as members of the group practice. Also, there are very strong incentives in training, in ethics, in liabilities, and in peer review situations that tend to make physicians very conservative about doing things they shouldn't do.

Frederick Rice*

Another disadvantage is the fact that the capitation system involves a substantial risk, particularly for the physician who unwittingly attracts a patient group with higher-than-average use of services. Of course, the HMO will provide some sort of cushion to prevent disastrous loss, and there is also a corresponding potential for financial gain. But because physicians are not used to assuming any risk other than that of bad debt, they may be reluctant to join such a program. This may magnify far the direct capitation HMO the tradeoff between the amount of risk it is able to transfer to the physician and the relative ease with which it can persuade physicians to participate.

Despite the disadvantages, the flexibility of this third type of HMO makes it an attractive approach for use in metropolitan areas with large numbers of physicians. Like other models, this HMO can select physicians already using fewer-than-average services per patient while delivering high-quality medical care, and thereby reduce operating costs. But this model's individual rather than pooled risk should also attract physicians whose practice patterns are economical.

The direct capitation system may also be a useful model for an in-house HMO. If the company has access to the claims data for its employees, it can determine which of the physicians used by the employees appear to be prime candidates for capitation agreements. By concentrating on those physicians already used by its employees, the company minimizes employee resistance to a "company plan."

Potential Partners for HMO Development

The focus of this chapter has been on the physician component of an HMO. Another consideration in an HMO development effort is whether the sponsor should look for co-sponsors from among major consumer groups in the community, particularly other large employers or unions; hospitals; insurance carriers, including Blue Cross, Blue Shield, and commercial carriers; and the federal government. As a general rule, the two advantages of partnership are provision of broader expertise to draw upon and more potential sources of start-up capital and HMO members. On the other hand, partners tend to reduce flexibility, increase the development time, and complicate the effort if the partners have different interests. The partnership issue is also one of timing: at

*Executive Director, Valley Health Plan, Amherst, Massachusetts.

what point in the development process does an industry "go public" with its plans for an HMO? This was discussed briefly in chapter 2.

Potential partners with the most consonant interests are other companies or unions in the area. Examples of this kind of joint sponsorship are the Greater Delaware Valley Health Care, Inc., an HMO sponsored by local companies, the Twin City Health Care Development Project, where twenty companies formed an organization to promote HMO development, and the Rhode Island Group Health Association, founded by an AFL-CIO State Council.[20] While all of these partnerships were successful, each discovered the importance of obtaining the commitment of the top levels of their various member organizations to the project.

Efforts at joint sponsorship of an HMO in Winston-Salem, North Carolina were less satisfactory. One company participant, R. J. Reynolds, grew impatient with the slow pace of development and decided to go ahead on its own. This led to the rapid and successful development of a salaried group HMO, as described earlier in this chapter.

The decision whether or not to bring in corporate partners hinges on two questions. First, how much clout does the initiating company have in the area? If the dominant employer has decided to embark on an HMO development effort, it can probably do so without having to turn to other companies for assistance. On the other hand, if the area is without a dominant employer, as is the Delaware Valley in Pennsylvania, then a cooperative effort may be needed to insure sufficient support.

Second, is the goal to sponsor an HMO or to encourage HMO development? The latter goal, exemplified by the Twin City Project, entails a pluralistic system comprised of several HMOs. Such an effort would almost certainly be beyond the capabilities of any one company in a metropolitan area. On the other hand, direct sponsorship of one HMO, with a company's own work force as the primary market, would be practical for a company with a sufficient number of employees. Some large employers may even opt for an in-house HMO.

A company or union may also choose to work with other consumer groups in the community. In the case of the Twin City Project, broad community representation was desirable since it aided in the acceptance of the HMO concept by the community at large. Again, the question of joint sponsorship hinges on a trade-off between bringing aboard all parties whose support will eventually be required for successful operation, and possible loss of control and flexibility in the development process because of multiple sponsors with varying interests.

The hospital community is another possible source for partners. Clearly, the HMO must work with at least a subset of the hospital community if it is to deliver its product. But the HMO developer has considerable flexibility in the determination of when and how to bring the hospital community into the HMO process, depending on the type of HMO being planned.

There are essentially three levels of hospital involvement possible in an HMO. The first is full partnership, in which the hospital(s) puts up part of the capital and/or shares in some part of the risk of providing hospital services. Full partnership is likely whenever the HMO is based on a component of the hospital, such as a hospital-based group practice or an IPA based on a hospital medical staff. However, hospital partnership may also become a part of any other HMO design. For example, many existing multispecialty group practices admit most of their patients to one hospital, and thus may wish to bring that hospital in as a partner at the beginning of the HMO development process.

The advantages of having a hospital as a full partner, in addition to the funds and expertise it can provide, are that the HMO will be assured access to needed hospital beds and can sometimes obtain a discount on room rates for its members. The access issue is particularly acute for new salaried group HMOs, which often bring in new physicians with no established privileges at local hospitals. Since the granting of hospital privileges is usually the province of the medical staff, some salaried group HMOs have had problems in areas where the medical staffs opposed the growth of these HMOs. For example, the Harvard Community Health Plan's expansion plans have been delayed by its difficulties in obtaining hospital bed commitments from some hospitals.

The price break obtained from a hospital partnership can take a variety of forms. The hospital may agree to accept a capitation payment for the provision of all hospital services to HMO members, and thus accept part of the risk of providing these services. The three hospitals participating in the Greater Delaware Valley Health Plan have agreed to such an arrangement. This kind of hospital capitation payment is usually subject to a ceiling on total use of the hospital, since the hospital does not control the behavior of the physicians who decide on hospitalization. The more common arrangement is for the hospital to agree to provide services at a discount, which usually means providing them at, or slightly above, cost.

The disadvantage of company-hospital partnership is that the partners have conflicting interests. A major goal of the corporate developer is to reduce hospital utilization, which strikes at the financial viability of the hospital. Thus, the hospital's interests, if narrowly defined, may not be served by a successful HMO. However, from a broader perspective, if the community has an excess of hospitals and beds, then by co-sponsoring an HMO, the hospital can hope to increase its market share in order to offset the lower hospitalization rate. Or, if the hospital receives a share of the surpluses generated through reduced hospitalization, it can use those funds to adapt to changing circumstances by reducing the number of beds and altering the services it offers. Hospitals are thus beginning to face the problems posed to them by HMO development:

> It is true that HMOs contribute to the decline in hospital utilization rates and that, therefore, some hospitals may go out of business. This is already happening and may be necessary to solve some of the health care problems. It should be noted, however, that the HMO is one of many influences affecting hospital viability. Recognizing all of the above, the Massachusetts Hospital Association is supportive of HMOs. The philosophy of an HMO is compatible with the ideals hospital administrators have been taught, that is, quality care for the lowest possible cost.
>
> Jocelyn Carlson*

*Vice President for Professional and Community Services, Massachusetts Hospital Association.

In the city of Wausau there were two hospitals at the time that we started, with a total of 410 beds. About 1971 the two merged and planned for a new hospital of 500 beds. The hospital is now being built; it's going to open in early 1979—but with 264 beds.

Jacob J. Spies

At the second level of hospital involvement in an HMO, the latter contracts for services with a subset of the available hospitals. This is probably the most common type of hospital-HMO relationship. Again, the HMO usually gives the contracting hospitals all of its hospital business in exchange for hospital privileges and perhaps a discount. The arrangements are generally similar to those described above, except that the hospitals are less likely to bear a share of the risk. The most common arrangement, used by the Health Maintenance Organization of Pennsylvania and the Southshore Health Plan (case 9), is to pay a rate based on the Blue Cross rate, instead of full charges. The kind of bargain that can be struck will depend on the potential size of the HMO, both in terms of total members and market share, and on the competitive framework of the hospital community, which will be a function of the amount of existing overcapacity.

The third level involves loose or indirect (third-party) contracts between the HMO and the hospitals. The HMO either agrees to pay full hospital charges or purchases hospital coverage through a third party, usually Blue Cross, and relies on the contracts between the third party and the hospitals. While this would entail the HMO paying some additional charge to cover the third party's overhead, it may be attractive to a small HMO since it could avoid setting up its own system for paying hospital claims.

Another source of partners is the health insurance industry. Insurers can bring to a partnership considerable experience in marketing, claims processing, and management information systems, as well as considerable capital. The Blue Cross plans, Employers Insurance of Wausau, the Prudential Insurance Company of America and the Connecticut General Life Insurance Company have been among the more active health insurers in HMO development. In general, though, active intervention in the health care system is still a relatively recent phenomenon in the health insurance industry:

People have asked us, as insurers with so much purchasing power in health care, "Why haven't you been able to do more in the area of cost containment?" One, we haven't been asked to. The people we have to be responsible to first and foremost are policyholders and beneficiaries. And until the cost crunch of the last few years, none of the policyholders have wanted to buy cost containment features in their plan, and none have really asked us about it.

J. David Seay*

An approach to carrier partnership in an HMO is for the carrier to do the marketing and enrollment, develop the management information system, and pay for certain parts of the benefit package, such as emergency care, out-of-area coverage, reinsurance, and, particularly in cases where Blue Cross is a partner,

*Staff Executive, Group Operations, John Hancock Mutual Life Insurance Company.

CASE 9

Southshore Health Plan

HMO Type: Fee-for-service IPA

Location: Atlantic County, New Jersey

Original sponsor(s): Physicians

Starting date: September 1977

Service area population: 200,000

Enrollment: 1,600

Participating physicians: 107

In 1971, a small number of physicians in the greater Atlantic City area of New Jersey confronted the problems of a
rapidly increasing elderly and poor population, a declining
number of practicing physicians, especially in primary care, and
the need for improvements in the health delivery system as reflected by very poor local public health statistics. At first, the
physicians planned to establish a medical group model HMO,
and in 1972 a grant was obtained from HEW for the project.
However, the realities of the situation, including a lack of interest in abrupt shifts in practice style among the established and
busy physician community, the dispersed nature of the population, and the limited group market available, quickly dampened
enthusiasm for this approach. Therefore, the project initiators
decided to develop a fee-for-service type of HMO in response to
the continuing community and physician concerns about the
availability, continuity, and cost of health care.

Federal funding was secured to develop a fee-for-service
IPA-HMO, and continued through June 1976. However, the federal government questioned the plan's ability to enroll a break-
even membership in a community with a marginal group market
and fairly low health insurance benefits. As a result, Southshore
was denied qualification, making the plan ineligible for federal
loans needed to begin operations and offset initial operating deficits. Rather than disband, the plan's board of directors invited
the Prudential Insurance Company of America to undertake
management, financing, and marketing of the program. After
performing its own review of the plan's feasibility, Prudential
decided that a somewhat streamlined approach, having a lower

break-even enrollment, would be possible. State approval of the revised program was obtained, and the HMO opened in September 1977. Southshore submitted a second application for federal qualification in mid-1978; it is now pending.

The nonprofit Southshore Health Plan has a board of directors representing community interests, including physicians, members (consumers), and nonphysician providers. Prudential is responsible for providing staff to manage the program. Under the terms of the HMO's contract with the IPA, the HMO establishes an account to cover physician claims by transferring a monthly capitation for each HMO member to the IPA. Separate accounts are established and maintained by the HMO for hospital claims and for emergency room and laboratory claims. The IPA account sets an upper limit on the funds available to meet physician claims, subject to possible physician sharing of savings realized by controlling hospital, laboratory, and emergency room utilization. Participating physicians draw on this physician account by submitting claims for services rendered to HMO members. Approved claims are paid on a fee-for-service basis up to the physician's usual and customary fee, within the limits of a maximum fee schedule, and subject to a 20 percent hold back. If physician claims exceed budgeted levels, they are paid out of the reserve created by the withheld fees. If dollars remain in the physician fund at year's end, the HMO uses them to meet a portion of any deficit in the hospital or emergency room and laboratory accounts. If there are surpluses in the HMO's accounts for hospital or emergency room/laboratory services, an agreed-upon portion of those surpluses is credited to the physician account. After this year-end settlement process, any positive balance in the physician fund is distributed to the participating physicians.

The HMO contracts with the two local hospitals, and pays them an inclusive per diem rate based upon each hospital's requested Blue Cross rate. Utilization is budgeted at 600 days per 1,000 members annually, and the program uses a stringent package of utilization controls, including preadmission certification of nonemergency cases, and referral controls requiring authorization by the primary care physician of visits to referral physicians and hospital admissions recommended by referral physicians. During the program's first ten months of operation, annualized hospital utilization was approximately 500 days per 1,000 members. Thus far, marketing has been complicated by the false start in 1976 and the lack of federal qualification, but the plan is meeting its enrollment projections.

Sources

James Brittain, Executive Director, Southshore Health Plan, personal communication, July and August 1978.

Betsy Ann Rogge, Medical Services Coordinator, Southshore Health Plan,
personal communication, May 1978.

Victor Bressler, "The Southshore Health Plan: An Example of an Open-
Panel HMO," in HMO/IPA, How Will It Affect Me? (Trenton, New
Jersey: New Jersey Foundation for Health Care Evaluation, 1977), pp.
83–89.

Plan materials: "Brief History of Southshore Health Plan," and Physician's
Provider Handbook (Northfield, New Jersey: Southshore Health Plan).

---

hospitalization coverage. Examples include the North Central Health Protection Plan and the Greater Marshfield Community Health Plan, both in Wiscon-
sin. The various kinds of coverage are usually provided through an ex-
perience-rated insurance policy purchased by the HMO from the carrier.
Obviously, such an arrangement helps lower the development and overhead
costs of the HMO, which can be critical for successful implementation of the
HMO. As another example of what a carrier can do for a developing HMO, the
Prudential Life Insurance Company manages both a salaried group HMO, the
Rhode Island Group Health Association, and a fee-for-service HMO, South-
shore Health Plan, under contract.

The major potential problem associated with carrier partnership, or use of
a carrier to provide such central services as marketing, is that the carrier's
interests do not necessarily correspond to those of the HMO. The problem of
divergent interests will be acute where the carrier already has a significant
market share, and thus must cannibalize its own subscribers to provide the
HMO with members.

Another problem related to carrier marketing is that the carrier often
expects its current sales force to do the marketing. Since the HMO is a new and
unfamiliar product for this sales force, and often one that does not yield the
same financial rewards as traditional policy sales, the sales force has not always
done a very effective job. This was a major problem with the initial marketing
effort undertaken by Blue Cross/Blue Shield of Massachusetts for the Harvard
Community Health Plan. Experience indicates that a carrier should create a
special sales group to market the HMO and devote sufficient resources to the
effort to insure success.

Thus, the decision whether or not to use carrier partnership will often
hinge on the degree of commitment by the carrier to the success of the HMO:

We sought to strike a deal with Blue Shield and Blue Cross of
Massachusetts and were subjected to one time delay after another.
The initial enrollment estimate of 50,000 people sounded great; all

of a sudden, it dropped to 2,500, and the commitment of the traditional insurance carriers became more and more of a concern to the physician community. We finally came across Frank B. Hall & Company, which was willing to front-end—to the tune of $250,000—the development of a complete marketing strategy, sales promotional campaign, brochures, and so on.

Gary Janko

We have three and one-half million members and ready access to the market in Massachusetts. Our representatives are on a first-name basis with key personnel in most of the industrial groups. We think we can offer a lot to any provider group, whether it be a hospital, a physician group practice, or a foundation for medical care. We bring in a commitment to HMOs and a marketing force that is second to none.

Richard Napolitano*

The last potential partner we will discuss is the federal government. The recently reorganized Office of Health Maintenance Organizations in the Department of Health, Education, and Welfare can provide funding to develop an HMO, and subsequently make loans and loan guarantees to operating plans. It also gives an HMO the advantage of mandatory dual choice for marketing. In return, the HMO has to meet the many requirements of the HMO Act and its attendant regulations, and must become qualified. In addition, the Office of Health Maintenance Organizations can provide technical assistance in developing HMOs, although the extent to which it will do so for HMOs which do not intend to seek qualification is as yet unclear.

There are problems associated with developing a federally qualified HMO. The HMO Act restricts the structure of the HMO to one of three models: the salaried group-staff model, the salaried group-medical group model, and the IPA.[21] Qualified HMOs are required to meet certain requirements, in terms of benefit package and community rating, which can weaken their ability to compete. Also, qualified HMOs must meet extensive reporting requirements which have been burdensome for many of the smaller plans. The Office of Health Maintenance Organizations is making a concerted effort to reduce these burdens, but accepting federal funds is always likely to mean accepting restrictions.

Even those plans which choose to proceed without federal support should probably be designed with qualification in mind. Except for in-house plans, it will be in the long-term best interest of the HMO to seek federal qualification at some point when it can meet federal requirements without threatening its own viability. Qualified plans now receive preferential treatment under the federal health planning law and are the only HMOs which can enroll Medicare and Medicaid recipients on a capitation, as opposed to a cost, basis. This is likely to be carried over into any national health insurance plan, which means that an HMO must be able to qualify in order to protect itself, should a national plan become a reality.

---

* Director of Health Planning and Development, Blue Shield of Massachusetts.

Furthermore, the federal government can be the source of enrollees for an HMO. The Federal Employees Health Benefits Program contracts with many HMOs around the country, and federal employees often constitute one of the largest membership groups for an HMO. The Federal Employees Health Benefits Program is also experimenting with HMO networks, within which several HMOs of the same type, either salaried group or fee-for-service, contract jointly with the program, charge one premium, and guarantee portability of coverage from one plan in the network to another. The Blue Cross Association is the coordinator of the salaried group HMO network, while the American Association of Foundations for Medical Care is the coordinator of the fee-for-service HMO network.

The federal government can also offer an HMO the opportunity to enroll Medicare and Medicaid recipients. While the ground rules for such contracts are still undergoing change, there is considerable interest on the part of both federal and state governments in enrolling these recipients in HMOs:

> We would like to see as many Medicaid recipients enrolled in HMOs as possile. The costs for the Harvard Community Health Plan currently are approximately 20 percent below the average fee-for-service expenditure for the average Medicaid recipient. But we do not want to see HMOs developing with only a Medicaid population or with a majority of Medicaid enrollees, because we know that the experiences in other states have been very adverse with respect to that.
>
> Joel Abrams*

Decisions concerning partnership—whether to seek partners and, if so, which ones to seek—will inevitably depend on individual circumstances. The initial sponsor, either company or union, will need to analyze this question along the following lines. How will the development process be financed? If the initial sponsor's resources are not sufficient, where is the best place to seek additional support? Will the proposed medical delivery system for the HMO require that the hospitals be an integral part of the process? Does the sponsor possess, or can it purchase, the necessary expertise to develop and run an HMO? Will it be necessary to involve other sponsors to give the HMO a reasonable chance to be successful in the marketplace? The answers to these questions will help resolve the issue of partnership.

Similarly, the selection of an HMO model for development in a given community will depend in part on characteristics of the company's work force and the size and composition of the community. Is the work force stable and thus likely to have established physician relationships, or is it growing rapidly? Do new employees complain about the difficulty of locating a family physician? Do the employees tend to live near the company, or are they widely scattered throughout a metropolitan area? Is the community fairly small, with only one or two hospitals, or is it a large city with many medical facilities? Finally, the wide variation in physician components that we have

*Director, Bureau of Community and Non-Institutional Services, Massachusetts Rate Setting Commission; Chairman, Massachusetts HMO Task Force.

explored in this chapter makes an analysis of the physician community a necessity. Do many of the physicians in the community practice in large multispecialty or family/general practice groups? Or do they tend to practice individually or in single specialty groups? Is the physician community part of one cohesive organization, such as the county medical society? Do the physicians tend to identify more strongly with a particular hospital than with the medical society? Are there identifiable leaders among community physicians? By answering such questions, the corporate sponsor can identify those HMO models which offer the best prospect for success in the particular area.

NOTES

1. Richard H. Egdahl, John Friedland, Anthony J. Mahler, and Diana Chapman Walsh, "Fee-for-Service HMOs," *Journal of the American Medical Association* (in press).

2. These figures are based on our review of the operations of various HMOs throughout the United States.

3. Robert G. Shouldice and Katherine H. Shouldice, *Medical Group Practice and Health Maintenance Organizations* (Washington, D.C.: Information Resources Press, 1978).

4. Louis J. Goodman, Edward H. Bennett III, and Richard J. Odem, "Current Status of Group Medical Practice in the United States," *Public Health Reports* 92 (5) (September–October 1977): 430–443 (hereafter, *Current Status*).

5. Cecil C. Cutting, "Historical Development and Operating Concepts," in *The Kaiser Permanente Medical Care Program: A Symposium*, Anne R. Somers, ed. (New York: The Commonwealth Fund, 1971), pp. 17–22.

6. Bynum E. Tudor, "A New Corporate Prepaid Group Health Plan," in *Background Papers on Industry's Changing Role in Health Care Delivery*, Richard H. Egdahl, ed., Springer Series on Industry and Health Care, No. 3 (New York: Springer-Verlag, 1977), pp. 70–78.

7. Joseph L. Dorsey, "Prepaid Group Practice and the Delivery of Ambulatory Care," *New England Journal of Medicine 291* (7) (August 15, 1974): 361–363.

8. John R. Kress and James Singer, *HMO Handbook* (Rockville, Maryland: Aspen Systems Corporation, 1975), p. 110.

9. Aaron Wildavsky, "Doing Better and Feeling Worse: The Political Pathology of Health Policy," *Daedalus, Journal of the American Academy of Arts and Sciences* (Winter, 1977): 105–123.

10. Harold S. Luft, "How do Health-Maintenance Organizations Achieve Their Savings?" *New England Journal of Medicine, 298* (24) (June 15, 1978): 1336–1343.

11. Lawrence G. Goldberg and Warren Greenberg, "Staff Report on the Health Maintenance Organization and its Effects on Competition" (Washington, D.C.: Federal Trade Commission, Bureau of Economics, July 1977).

12. Seymour Lusterman, *Industry Roles in Health Care* (New York: The Conference Board, 1974), p. 83.

13. *Current Status*, p. 431.

14. Ibid., p. 440. This count includes a number of medical groups which were created for new salaried group HMOs.

15. Richard H. Egdahl, et al., "The Potential of Organizations of Fee-for-Service Physicians for Achieving Significant Decreases in Hospitalization," *Annals of Surgery, 186* (1977): 156–167.

16. Jacob J. Spies, "A Corporation's Experience with Independent Practice Association HMOs," in *Background Papers on Industry's Changing Role in Health Care Delivery*, Richard H. Egdahl, ed., Springer Series on Industry and Health Care, No. 3 (New York: Springer-Verlag, 1977), pp. 3–15.

17. Lloyd Mathwick and Anthony Masso, "The New Mexico Health Care Corporation: A Discussion of the First Two Years of Operation," (Rockville, Maryland and Albuquerque, New Mexico: Department of Health, Education, and Welfare, Health Services Administration, Bureau of Community Health Services, Health Maintenance Organizations, and The New Mexico Health Care Corporation, April 15, 1975).

18. Remarks by Alfred F. Dougherty, Jr., Director, Bureau of Competition, Federal Trade Commission, at the National Health Lawyers Association Seminar on Antitrust in the Health Care Field, Washington, D.C., December 13, 1977.

19. Alain C. Enthoven, "Shattuck Lecture—Cutting Cost Without Cutting the Quality of Care," *New England Journal of Medicine*, 298 (22) (June 1, 1978): 1229–1238.

20. Remarks by Edwin C. Brown, Secretary-Treasurer, Rhode Island AFL-CIO, and President, Rhode Island Group Health Association, at the Secretary's National HMO Conference, Washington, D.C., March 10, 1978.

21. Some direct capitation model HMOs can also qualify as IPAs if they meet the organizational requirements; e.g., HMO of Pennsylvania.

Assessing Legal Obstacles

John D. Blum

The purpose of this chapter is to evaluate some of the legal issues underlying corporate sponsorship of an HMO. These include common areas of HMO liability, the potential for corporate liability, the role of state law in regulating HMOs, the effects of the Employee Retirement Income Security Act (ERISA), and the antitrust implications of corporate-sponsored HMOs.

Liability Issues for the HMO

In reviewing the potential liability problems that a prepaid health plan could face, the areas of malpractice, due process, and confidentiality emerge as key concerns. The experiences of operating HMOs suggest that legal liability will not be as significant a problem for a prepaid health plan as it has been in other sectors of the health care delivery system.[1] Still, within the HMO there are potential areas of risk that could generate legal actions for malpractice, violation of procedural rights, or breach of confidentiality. Companies considering HMO sponsorship should be aware of the unique effects these legal issues may have on a prepaid health care plan.

Malpractice

In any medical practice setting, it can be expected that some errors of act or omission will occur that are of such a nature as to constitute actionable negligence. In an HMO providing a wide variety of medical services, the possibility of malpractice would seem to be great. In fact, however, HMOs have a lower rate of liability actions than other health provider organizations.[2]

HMOs have several built-in factors which minimize the potential for medical liability. First, prepayment offers participating physicians an incentive to avoid unnecessary treatment, thereby generally reducing liability exposure. Careful selection of participating physicians, utilization review, and quality assurance are all activities regularly conducted by HMOs which lower the organizational vulnerability to liability suits. Another significant factor in reducing potential negligence is the use of complaint or grievance mechanisms for HMO enrollees. Some states, such as California, require HMOs to establish grievance procedures. Even where malpractice claims cannot be handled through an internal grievance mechanism, such procedural devices help settle enrollee complaints at an early stage, before they mature into legal actions. State legislation has been enacted to exempt HMOs from malpractice liability.[3] In Illinois, for example, there is a statute which exempts medical service plan corporations from liability for medical negligence committed by plan physicians.[4] However, in light of recent developments in the area of corporate malpractice, there is some doubt that laws exempting HMOs from liability would be upheld in court.

The key question in regard to malpractice is whether the HMO corporation can be held legally responsible for the malpractice of its physician members. It is important to note that the potential for negligence will vary depending on the organizational structure of the HMO.

In an IPA, or open panel, model, the potential for liability is affected by whether the physician component is a separate corporation. If an IPA is an independent entity, the HMO management corporation is probably liable only for failure to ensure that qualified physicians are hired by the IPA. The IPA corporation, on the other hand, could be sued for physician member negligence, although the chances of such a suit succeeding would be questionable. The IPA is a corporate entity whose primary purpose is to have its members deliver services to HMO enrollees (as well as to monitor utilization and quality); as such, it is not a direct medical service provider. The IPA is primarily liable with respect to the competency of its member physicians and the adequacy of its monitoring devices.

In a situation where the IPA and HMO constitute one corporation instead of separate entities, liabilities cannot be divided between management and professional services, and the entity is thus more vulnerable to suit for medical negligence. If the IPA is a specialty or multispecialty group that, as a corporation, is directly involved in the delivery of services, the nature of its liability changes; in this case, the IPA has the same potential liability as any other health service provider organization.

A salaried group (closed panel) HMO, in which physicians are employed by the plan or are under contract to it, bears a greater degree of liability than an IPA. The closed panel is analogous to a hospital corporation, whose liability in some jurisdictions has been extended to cover the quality of medical services provided in the institution.[5] While physicians on hospital medical staffs have been traditionally viewed as independent contractors, that status is starting to change.[6] Physician groups which provide services exclusively to a hospital under contract have been viewed for purposes of liability as falling within the master-servant doctrine (respondeat superior). It can be argued that the salaried group HMO which provides medical services similar to those provided in a hospital should be held responsible under the common law for the quality of care delivered through its auspices. Further, if the respondeat superior doctrine is applicable to physicians under contract to provide a given service to a hospital, there is no reason why that doctrine could not be extended to a physician (or group) providing medical services to an HMO.

Procedural Fairness

An important issue related to the organizational liability of an HMO is the reduction of privileges or removal of a physician from a particular plan. Under statutory law and, to a lesser extent, under common law, the HMO has a duty to monitor the quality of medical care it provides, and it must take action against a participating physician whose performance has not been satisfactory. In carrying out any type of corrective or disciplinary action, HMO management must be cognizant of the rights of the individual physician. Improper sanction could lead to liability based on an action for violation of procedural due process of law rights.[7] Prior to removing or suspending a physician from the plan, the HMO must notify the individual of the charges and the right to a hearing. It is of critical importance that the HMO have adequate evidence prior to taking action against a participating physician, and that it keep accurate records of all proceedings. The number of procedural steps taken in a disciplinary case will be contingent, at least in part, on the course of action contemplated by the HMO against the practitioner.

Procedural due process is a constitutional doctrine and, as such, is not applicable to purely private entities.[8] In the hospital area, for example, courts regularly refuse to consider due process challenges where there is no governmental involvement or state action. Even where state action exists, courts often review only the adequacy of a given disciplinary system and not the merits of the particular action. An HMO which is strictly a private entity would thus not be subject to constitutional challenge for a procedural due process violation. Those plans that are federally qualified, however, may have sufficient governmental contact, by virtue of funding and regulation to classify their behavior as state action. It should be noted that in some jurisdictions the concept of due process has been replaced by that of fairness, in order to circumvent the artificialities of constitutional law.[9] Under this doctrine of fundamental fairness derived from the common law, a health care institution is seen as operating in the public interest; failure to afford a physician fair treatment prior to dismissal is interpreted as an illegal violation of the public interest.

Confidentiality

The issue of personal privacy in medical treatment has received increased attention with the growth of large-scale record-keeping systems in both the public and private sectors. While the law concerning medical privacy has expanded, by and large, the confidentiality of personal medical records is still linked to the physician-patient privilege, which requires that information a patient passes on to a physician, or which is developed in the course of treatment, be held in confidence.[10] The privilege has been recognized as falling within the ambit of constitutional protection, and it has been legislated as a protected right in many states.

In assessing the confidentiality policies of an HMO, both common and statutory law come into play. The common law physician-patient privilege would clearly be applicable to the relationship between a physician and an enrollee in an HMO. However, it seems unreasonable to argue that because the prepaid plan offers comprehensive medical services, the ambit of the physician-patient relationship should be expanded to include the HMO as a whole. On the statutory side, there are a number of state laws which require HMOs to treat patient records as confidential.[11] For example, according to the health maintenance provisions of the State of New York, "unless the patient waives the right of confidentiality, an HMO or its comprehensive health services plan shall not be allowed to disclose any information which was acquired by such organization or plan in the course of the rendering to a patient of professional services."[12] The Colorado HMO law actually extends the physician-patient privilege to include the entire HMO organization.[13]

Patient confidentiality can be protected by means of a clause in the enrollment contract specifying that personal medical data will be handled confidentially. Where confidentiality is not specified, it could be argued that the HMO has an implied or quasicontractural obligation to protect patient privacy.[14] However, absolute protection of patient data is neither possible nor practical within the HMO organization. Prepaid plans may require enrollees to grant the organization a waiver to allow use of patient data for internal quality review, research, billing, etc. Also, the HMO cannot guarantee protection of medical records from subpoena under state evidence law. Finally, disclosure of patient data may be necessary for medical reasons.

Corporations sponsoring HMOs should not pressure these organizations to release identifiable medical data on company employees. Undue pressure from corporate sponsors would force the HMOs to compromise their confidentiality policies and would expose them to liability. Aggregate data, in all but the most unusual cases, should be sufficient to monitor corporate investment in a particular plan.

The HMO must also be concerned with protecting information concerning the practices of physician members. Whether they actually store medical records or only obtain information from claims forms, HMOs require practice data for legal, administrative, and medical purposes. It is common for HMOs to develop practice profiles on individual physician members to evaluate the type of care they are providing for enrollees. While such physician data are critical for internal operations, they are not subject to disclosure except when mandated by federal or state law.[15] It would be highly unusual for an HMO to release physician member data without express permission or under a statutory mandate.

Apart from statutory grounds, a physician could challenge a prepaid plan for unauthorized disclosure under the tort doctrine of privacy.[16] A more likely cause of action against an HMO for unauthorized release of physician data is breach of contract. The physician-plan agreement may actually specify, if not imply, that the HMO will protect personally identifiable physician data.

Physician practice profiles developed by a prepaid health plan can raise interesting questions regarding confidentiality. Profiles that represent a pattern of behavior over time could be used as valuable evidence in a malpractice action against both the physician member and the HMO. Even if the rules of evidence precluded use of such profiles in court, they could prove valuable for purposes of pretrial discovery. Physicians in prepaid plans may be protected from subpoena of profile data under state law. Many states have statutes which safeguard the records and documents of medical quality assurance boards from subpoena for use in trial or discovery proceedings.[17] Since physician profiles are likely to be developed as part of an HMO's quality assurance program, their confidentiality will be protected in those states which have passed such statutes.

Corporate Liability

Although tort liability has not proven a serious problem for HMOs, corporations must be concerned about whether they can be held legally accountable for negligence occurring in plans that they sponsor. Under well-established principles of corporate law, a parent company is generally not liable for the torts of a subsidiary corporation.[18] There are instances, however, when a corporation will be held liable for the legal wrongs of a subsidiary. Determination of a parent company's liability is usually based on consideration of such factors as funding support, overlap of corporate directors and officers, and ability of the subsidiary to act independently.[19] If enough control is exerted by the parent corporation, a court may choose to ignore the corporate status of a subsidiary and attribute liability directly to the founding entity.

A nonprofit HMO sponsored by a corporation is not a subsidiary, but the applicable corporate liability principles are not necessarily limited to a subsidiary company. A Texas federal district court, in *Bay Sound Transportation Company v. U.S.*,[20] upheld what it classified as a well-established rule that one corporation exerting control over a second will be liable for the torts of the second entity. It was not specified that the controlled corporation must be a subsidiary.

If it can be shown that an HMO is completely dominated by the corporate sponsor, negligence in the prepaid plan may be attributed to the sponsoring company. Factors influencing the determination of corporate liability for an HMO would include eligibility requirements (i.e., whether the plan is open to groups other than the employees of the sponsor), the amount of capital support provided, the number of corporate representatives on the HMO board, and the extent of overall integration between the HMO and the corporate sponsor's business interests. In carrying out its function of delivering health services to corporate employees, the prepaid plan can be viewed as a type of controlled agent fulfilling a contractual duty held by the corporation. Under the agency theory, the company is liable for the negligent actions of its agents carried out for its own benefit.[21]

It does not always follow that, where one corporation has control over another, the party with the controlling interest will be held liable for all the torts of the controlled entity. The activity on which liability is based must further the corporate interest and be an area over which the corporation has control.[22] Thus, even if it can be demonstrated that an HMO is totally controlled by the corporate sponsor, the sponsor will not be held liable for all negligent occurrences, but only those in which a controlling factor is shown.

A major concern in considering potential corporate liability is medical malpractice, because it represents perhaps the most recognizable risk in any health care delivery system. The agency theory can be used to argue that the malpractice of HMO physicians should be attributed to the corporate sponsor. If the HMO is a corporate shell established to provide medical care to the company employees, the physicians in the HMO become agents of the corporation, carrying out the obligation of the company to provide medical services to its employees. The agency argument is easier to establish in the case of a salaried group HMO, where physicians are directly employed by or under contract to the HMO, than in the case of an IPA, where the physican group is a separate corporate entity, and therefore the ties of agency are not as direct.

Corporate liability for the negligence of physician employees or agents has generally been difficult to establish because physicians are traditionally characterized as independent contractors. However, recent court decisions have viewed company physicians as corporate agents fulfilling a contractual obligation of their employer and, as such, creating liability for the principal corporation.[23] Nevertheless, in the case of an HMO, the corporate entity must be completely negated before an agency relationship can be created between HMO physicians and the corporate sponsor.

In considering corporate liability for HMO negligence, the effect of workmen's compensation must be considered. HMO treatment of work-related ailments (which is now a broad category) is covered by workmen's compensation.[24] If malpractice in the HMO aggravates a work-related injury, workmen's compensation is usually an exclusive remedy to cover that episode, thus precluding suit against the corporation.[25]

It is also possible to hold a parent corporation liable for breach of contract by a subsidiary or controlled spin-off.[26] The establishment of a contractual obligation on the part of the parent corporation is based on demonstration of control over the subsidiary similar to that required in tort liability. It is clear from a reading of the cases in both the contract and tort field that, in order to pierce the corporate veil, it must be shown that dominance over a subsidiary's activities goes beyond one or two areas of operation.

A number of theories can serve as the basis for establishing the contract obligation of a parent company. The alter ego theory, the identity theory, and the instrumentality rule all focus on the degree to which the subsidiary is being used to foster the ends of the parent company.[27] Some courts require demonstration of moral culpability on the part of the controlling party before it can be held responsible for the contractual obligations of the controlled entity.[28] Two other theories which have been used to establish a contractual duty are the doctrines of agency and estoppel.[29] It is conceivable that one of these theories could be used to render a corporation liable for the contractual obligations of the sponsored HMO. Certainly, any of the contracts which an HMO enters into with providers, health care institutions, suppliers, and so forth could generate breach-of-contract suits against the corporate sponsor.

State Law

Both federal and state laws play a significant role in the creation and regulation of prepaid health care plans. Qualification under federal law, while not essential, may in fact be necessary for the viable operation of a new HMO. Much has been written about the various provisions of the federal HMO laws, particularly the dual-choice requirement. The role of state law in HMO development is also important, since all prepaid health care plans must be established under some type of state enabling legislation. Thus, HMO development should be preceded by a careful assessment of federal and state HMO legislation, as well as an understanding of the way in which these two bodies of law interact.

Under the federal HMO Act, state legislation which impedes the development of an HMO is preempted.[30] Federal preemption is not nearly as complete as initial impression may lead one to believe. Specifically, the preemption provision prevents states from requiring medical society approval of an HMO or requiring that a certain percentage of physicians in a given area belong to the HMO. In addition, states may not require that an HMO be financed as an insurance carrier and may not prohibit advertising.[31] Apart from these stipulations and the preemption of laws designed to thwart the federal HMO effort, states clearly have the ability to establish regulations affecting the creation, marketing practices, financial condition, and quality of medical care of a prepaid health care plan, even if it is federally qualified.

It should be noted that each state law contains provisions unique to a given jurisdiction, and HMO legislation can change frequently. As of this writing, thirty-two states have enabling legislation designed specifically for the creation and regulation of HMOs.[32] In those jurisdictions where no enabling legislation exists, HMOs can be established under insurance laws or nonprofit corporation statutes. While enabling legislation varies from one state to another, there are many similarities, since several of these statutes are based on a model act developed by the National Association of Insurance Commissioners.[33]

State laws generally split the licensing and regulatory functions in regard to prepaid health plans between insurance departments, which are concerned with the financial aspects of HMOs, and departments of public health, which monitor the quality of medical care. Two exceptions are California, where HMOs are regulated by the Corporation Commissioner,[34] and Oklahoma, where a health planning commission has primary authority over HMOs.[35] Most state laws place no limitation on prepaid plan sponsorship; both nonprofit and for-profit entities are allowed to develop plans. In the few jurisdictions where HMO enabling legislation does not cover for-profit arrangements, such entities can be incorporated under insurance laws. Only ten states have legislation which specifically authorizes the formation and operation of HMOs by Blue Cross/Blue Shield and other commercial insurance companies;[36] this does not preclude the health insurance firms in other states from various types of involvement with HMOs ranges from consulting support to reinsurance arrangements.

Some state statutes allow the regulatory authority broad power to monitor the fiscal soundness of a given plan.[37] Regulators are concerned with the amount of working capital an HMO has, backup arrangements in the event of insolvency, and the existence of appropriate surety devices. Several states have specific regulations that require the HMO either to deposit cash or securities with the insurance department, or to submit a surety bond to guarantee performance.[38] Surety and reserve requirements have been criticized on the grounds that they deter HMO formation and are inconsistent with the nature of a prepaid plan as a service organization.[39]

An important part of state HMO regulation deals with marketing disclosure requirements. Many states require that documents used by the HMO in dealing with subscribers (and potential subscribers), such as policy forms, must first be approved by the state to ensure that they are both clear and concise. Some HMO laws also stipulate that potential enrollees must be given a state-approved prospectus listing the HMO's services, benefits, and financial provisions.[40] Another requirement in some states is that subscribers be allowed access to official HMO reports, such as financial statements, growth figures, and consumer grievance statements.[41] A key concession made in state law involves HMO solicitation of enrollees. Until recently, it was illegal for health care professionals to solicit business. Even before changes in the law in the area of health professional advertising occurred, special exemptions were granted to HMOs allowing them to educate the public concerning their services through advertising.[42]

State HMO legislation is designed to influence, to varying degrees, the costs, quality, and availability of medical resources. In many jurisdictions HMOs are required to report utilization patterns to health departments as a means of drawing comparisons with the fee-for-service sector. HMOs are often mandated to establish quality assurance programs; in some instances, the state actively monitors the quality of care in prepaid plans. In Iowa, external peer review of HMOs is conducted by the state's Professional Standards Review Organization.[43]

State laws requiring coverage of routine inpatient and outpatient services in benefit packages are generally less extensive than federal requirements for

HMO coverage, thus allowing prepaid plans to compete with health insurers. In Kansas, for example, the medical services which must be covered by an HMO are determined by the Commissioner of Insurance on the basis of geographical availability.[44] At the other extreme, some states require extensive benefit packages, including such services as home health care,[45] vision care,[46] mental health treatment,[47] and comprehensive drug coverage.[48] However, the states must be careful not to require HMO benefit packages which are more extensive than federal requirements; if federally sponsored HMO development is hampered, state requirements may be subject to preemption.

In the area of rate regulation, the majority of state HMO acts provide for direct control of premiums. State insurance departments must approve HMO premiums to insure that rates are not excessive, inadequate, or discriminatory. This is similar to the regulation covering Blue Cross/Blue Shield rates. Critics have charged that HMO rate regulation should not be patterned after Blue Cross/Blue Shield requirements because of the considerable discrepancies in market power and the effect of minimum premium levels on HMO capital growth. In addition, regulation of Blue Cross/Blue Shield does not account for underlying provider costs.[49] However, it is generally recognized that some form of state HMO rate regulation is necessary as a means of guaranteeing financial solvency.

State laws, with few exceptions, do not require HMOs to institute special cost control measures. In only three states (Michigan, Minnesota, and South Dakota) must prepaid plans assume all the financial risk for covered services; however, many states require HMOs to contract for reinsurance. With the exception of California, state legislation does not encourage delegation of medical tasks to nonphysician health providers as a vehicle for reducing costs.[50] Even in California, where delegation is encouraged within the HMO, the ability to do so is limited by restrictions in the state's medical practice acts.

State laws attempting to influence availability of medical resources are not as strong as the federal law. Experience rating (as opposed to community rating) is permitted under state statutes, with provisions authorizing HMOs to charge different rates for different groups of enrollees. Some states require that prepaid plans conduct open enrollment after a certain period of operation, in some instances, after a shorter time than required by federal law.[51] Open enrollment provisions under state law apply to groups served by an HMO, but not necessarily to the community at large. Also, state HMO acts do not require that HMO enrollment be representative of the population. Provision of medical services to the elderly and the poor by a state-qualified HMO depends on the requirements of Medicare and Medicaid.

ERISA

The federal Employee Retirement Income Security Act of 1974 regulates the administration of private employee benefit and pension plans.[52] This statute exempts state laws regulating employee benefit plans with the exception of provisions dealing with workmen's compensation or disability insurance.[53] The problem faced by the HMO is whether or not, as a health service plan offered to employee groups, it can be classified as a type of welfare benefits plan under ERISA. If a prepaid health care plan is regulated by ERISA, it will have to comply with the statute's stringent reporting and fiduciary requirements. Thus, whether or not an HMO can be excluded from ERISA regulation may be a determining factor in corporate HMO sponsorship.

On March 10, 1978 a U.S. Labor Department press release took the position that federally qualified HMOs constitute a benefit and not a plan under ERISA.[54] ERISA is designed to affect employee welfare plans; it is not specifically geared toward controlling benefits offered under a health plan. The effect of the Labor Department position is to minimize the regulatory impact of ERISA on HMOs, although final determination of this issue rests with the federal courts. The fact that government policy classifies federally qualified HMOs as a benefit under ERISA should act as an incentive for prepaid plans to obtain federal qualification.

ERISA's impact on HMOs which have not received federal qualification is open to question. The issue of the ERISA exemption clause concerning state laws dealing with employee health benefit plans (some of which include HMO coverage) has been addressed in recent federal court actions. In the case of *Standard Oil Company of California v. Agsalud*,[55] a ninth circuit federal district court ruled that the ERISA exemption preempted the Hawaii Prepaid Health Care Act, which required that employers offer their employees a prepaid health care plan as part of the employee health benefit package. The court decided that a prepaid health care plan required under the Hawaii statute was a welfare benefits plan preempted by Section 514 of ERISA.[56] The court rejected the argument that the Hawaii statute was a social insurance law and, as such, was an exception to the ERISA exemption clause. In the words of the court:

> The Hawaii Act regulates a type of employee benefit plan generally and historically maintained for other reasons beyond workmen's and unemployment compensation and disability insurance. . . . By exempting only those plans maintained solely to comply with state social insurance laws Congress intended to make ERISA reach all types of plans not generally required by state law. In other words, Congress intended to permit only traditional forms of state social insurance laws to continue to operate and the Hawaii Act, the first state health insurance law in the country, is hardly a traditional social insurance law.[57]

Although federal court decisions concerning employee benefits reflect a definite tendency toward exemption of state law, so far only in the *Standard Oil* case has a court ruled that prepaid plans are covered by ERISA. In an action similar to the *Standard Oil* ruling, the ninth circuit federal court ruled in the case of *Hewlett-Packard v. Barnes* that the regulation of employee health benefit plans by California's Knox-Keene Law was a matter of ERISA and not state law jurisdiction.[58] The *Hewlett-Packard* decision did not, however, specify that an HMO was a plan for purposes of ERISA.

The *Standard Oil* case places in doubt the effect of state employer dual-choice requirements. State insurance laws which specify that employers must offer HMOs in their health benefit packages can be viewed as being preempted by ERISA. It should be noted that the ruling in *Standard Oil*, while important to similar actions, is not a precedent in other federal courts. It may be possible for states to encourage HMO development through health insurance laws or other types of legislation, without ERISA preemption. In any case, even if ERISA is not waived for state-approved, prepaid plans, employers can still realize substantial health care cost savings through HMO development.

Antitrust Law

The degree of scrutiny concerning potential antitrust violations in health care is increasing. Any corporation that enters into a relationship with a prepaid health care plan geared toward controlling medical costs must consider whether such action entails potential antitrust law violation.

HMO-corporate price agreements constitute the most obvious source of potential antitrust violation. Under Section One of the Sherman Antitrust Act, every contract, combination, or conspiracy in restraint of trade affecting interstate commerce is unlawful;[59] a price fixing violation is covered by this section or by a state law paralleling the federal statute. Only since the U.S. Supreme Court decision in the case of *Goldfarb v. Virginia State Bar*[60] have professional groups been subject to the Sherman Act.

Price fixing has been characterized by some courts as "per se" illegal, thus precluding any inquiry into the purpose or effect of the arrangement in question.[61] Clearly, not all situations where prices are set between parties constitute illegal price fixing. Although price negotiations between a large corporation and a new HMO may not be arms-length transactions, they do not necessarily constitute an attempt to fix medical fees. At worse, HMO-corporate price agreements may constitute an ancillary restraint of trade.

An ancillary restraint in a given arrangement is evaluated under the "rule of reason" and is judged lawful if the restraint is reasonable and necessary to the primary and legitimate purpose of the arrangement, and further, if it does not unreasonably affect competition and is not imposed by a party with monopoly power.[62] In the case of a corporate-HMO price agreement, such an arrangement is likely to be viewed as a reasonable way of stabilizing health care costs.

A corporation and a prepaid health plan can jointly develop a fee schedule without violation of antitrust law. There is nothing per se illegal about the use of fee schedules for evaluating the reasonableness of charges. It is possible, however, that a restraint of trade challenge can be raised if an HMO is pressured into developing a given fee schedule by a corporate purchaser. Fee schedules with express minimum limits raise potential antitrust problems, but schedules which allow for flexibility should withstand legal challenges.[63]

Another source of potential antitrust violation is the use of corporate purchasing power to limit competition, which is a form of monopoly, known as monopsony, violating Section Two of the Sherman Act.[64] In order for a corporate purchaser to be found guilty of monopsony, it must be demonstrated that the corporation has dominant market purchasing power. Where a company is the primary employer in a given area, its health care purchasing power has a significant impact on the local health care market. A company acquiring dominant health care purchasing power by establishing an HMO or by pressuring an established plan could use its market power to compel area physicians to participate in the plan or face loss of business. For example, the use of significant corporate market power is evident in the United Auto Workers' Union hearing aid benefit program.[65] Established in conjunction with the major automobile manufacturers in Michigan, this program potentially affects six million people. The legality of the hearing aid program is currently the subject of judicial action. Those challenging the program claim that the Union's dominant market power forces practitioners either to join under the reimbursement terms of the plan or to face loss of business in the area of auditory treatment.

Finally, it should be noted that monopsonistic power must be used coercively to constitute an antitrust law violation. If use of monopsonistic power results in the creation of an arrangement which does not preclude competition, whatever restraints exist may be considered reasonable.[66]

Any discussion of potential antitrust implications in HMO-corporation arrangements must take into account the effect of the McCarran-Ferguson Act.[67] Under this statute, whatever constitutes the "business of insurance" is exempt from the Sherman Act to the extent that it is governed by state law. It is not necessary that the state law regulate the particular activity in question; a general state regulatory scheme controlling insurance practices suffices for purposes of the McCarran-Ferguson Act.[68]

The key question that must be answered in any consideration of the McCarran-Ferguson Act is what constitutes the business of insurance. In this respect, prepaid health plans have received inconsistent treatment in the federal courts. In the case of *Manasen v. California Dental Services*,[69] which concerns an antitrust challenge against a prepaid dental plan, a federal district court ruled that the McCarran-Ferguson exemption was not limited to insurance companies but covered a range of activities affecting rate making, including settlement of claims and limitation of costs. The role of California Dental Services in setting the level of dental fees was recognized by the courts as being within the business of insurance, because it was a key factor in determining the cost of plan premiums, and thus the plan was ruled to be exempt from federal regulation.

In direct conflict with the *Manasen* decision is the fifth circuit case of *Royal Drug Co., Inc. v. Group Life & Health Insurance Co.*,[70] in which the court ruled that the pricing activities of a prepaid drug plan and a group of participating pharmacies did not fit within the business-of-insurance exemption. In disagreeing with *Manasen*, the court stated, "an activity is not part of the business of insurance solely because it has an impact, favorable or otherwise, upon premiums charged by the insurer." However, federal court decisions are generally in agreement with the *Manasen* ruling that the McCarran-Ferguson exemption should not be denied to professional service plans because they involve the delivery of products and services rather than indemnity.

The McCarran-Ferguson Act is not an absolute bar to antitrust coverage, since Section 3(b) of that law specifies an exception to the exemption provision for conduct which constitutes an unreasonable restraint of trade through boycott, coercion, or monopoly (in violation of the Sherman Act). In the recent U.S. Supreme Court decision in the case of *St. Paul Fire & Marine Insurance Co.*

v. Bary,[71] the court ruled that the exception was not limited to insurance company boycotts of agents and other insurance companies (which many federal courts have held), but that it included any act or agreement by an insurer amounting to boycott, coercion, or imitation. This case is significant for HMO-corporate cost control arrangements. If HMOs are found to be engaged in the business of insurance, they will not receive blanket protection under the McCarran-Ferguson Act if the agreements they develop with corporate sponsors place an unreasonable restraint of trade on a given medical community.

Conclusion

In evaluating the legal areas discussed above, ERISA and antitrust emerge as the most serious concerns for industry. While ERISA may be applicable to HMOs that are not federally qualified, it seems that the Department of Labor, in conjunction with HEW, can develop a regulatory scheme that would not significantly burden a prepaid health plan. The application of antitrust law to an HMO and its sponsor will be contingent on the market power that a given corporate purchaser has. The use of significant market power to control price and competition could lead to antitrust challenges, but only a handful of corporations appear to have the requisite purchasing power in a given market area.

As far as company sponsors being held liable for the negligence of HMOs is concerned, this is unlikely if corporations allow sponsored plans to operate independently. Corporations should not view the HMO as an extension of the corporate medical department. Those companies that become involved in the operation of an HMO may find themselves being held legally responsible for negligence occurring in the plan. It is especially important that corporations respect the confidentiality of employee medical records held by the HMO; these records should be shared only with company physicians when a worker's health so demands.

In assessing whether to become involved in HMO development, corporations cannot ignore potential legal problems. It does not seem, however, that the issues discussed herein pose insurmountable obstacles to HMO development. Corporate sponsors that are aware of legal pitfalls should be able to structure prepaid health plans and corporate involvement in those plans in such a way as to minimize legal difficulties.

NOTES

1. William J. Curran, George B. Moseley, "The Malpractice Experience of Health Maintenance Organizations," *Northwestern Law Review 70* (1975): 69.

2. Id.

3. Ill. State Corporations Chp. 32 § 589.

4. Id.

5. Arthur F. Southwick, George J. Siedel, *The Law of Hospital and Health Care Administration*, Chapter 12 (Ann Arbor, Michigan: Health Administration Press, 1978).

6. Id., p. 378.

7. John D. Blum, *Medical Discipline and Procedural Due Process: Evaluation of Hospital Staff Proceedings*, Part I, prepared for HEW Grant R01 HS 02044-01A1.

8. Robert J. Glennon, John E. Navak, "A Functional Analysis of the Fourteenth Amendment, 'State Action' Requirement," *The Supreme Court Review 1976*, p. 221.

9. John J. McMahon, "Judicial Review of Internal Policy Decisions of Private Nonprofit Hospitals: A Common Law Approach," *American Journal of Law & Medicine 3* (1977): 149.

10. 20 ALR3d 1109.

11. N.J.S.A. 26:2J-27.

12. N.Y. Public Health Law § 4410(2).

13. Colorado Revised Statutes § 10-17-127.

14. See *Horne v. Patten*, 287S.2d824 (Ala. 1974).

15. P.L. 92-603; see N.Y.S. Public Health Law §230(11).

16. William L. Prosser, *The Law of Torts*, Chapter 20, "Privacy" (St. Paul: West Publishing Co., 1971).

17. Erie W. Springer, "Professional Standards Review Organizations: Some Problems of Confidentiality," *Utah Law Review* 1975 (Summer): 361.

18. 7 ALR3d 1343.

19. Id.

20. 350 Fed. Supp. 420(1972).

21. Supra at n. 18.

22. Id.

23. John D. Blum, "Corporate Liability for Inhouse Medical Malpractice," *St. Louis University Law Journal 22*(1978).

24. Id.

25. Id.

26. 38 ALR3d 1102.

27. Id.

28. Id.

29. Id.

30. P.L. 93-222 § 1311.

31. Id.

32. Aspen Systems Corporation, *Health Maintenance Organization Laws: A National Overview*, prepared for DHEW, February 28, 1978.

33. National Association of Insurance Commissioners' Model Act (1972).

34. Cal. Health & Safety Code § 1341.

35. Okla. Stat. Ann. 63 § 2508.

36. For example, see Ark. Stat. Ann. §§ 66-5201-5228, Colorado Rev. Stat. Ann. §§ 10-17-104(2)(d).

37. See Cal. Health & Safety Code §1372.

38. See Colorado Rev. Stat. Ann. §§10-17-104(2)(d).

39. McNeil and Schlenker, "HMOs, Competition and Government," *Milbank Quarterly* 195 (1975): 207–208.

40. See S.C. Ins. Dept. Reg. R6-75 §5(j).

41. Several states make HMO filing reports part of the public domain following the National Association of Insurance Commissioners' Model Act.

42. See Nev. Rev. Stat. §695C.050(2).

43. Iowa Ins. Dept. Rule 12.5(11)(b)(1974).

44. Kan. Stat. Ann. §40-3202(f)(l)(Supp. 1975).

45. See Mich. Comp. Laws Ann. §325.903(2)(g)(1975).

46. Supra at n. 42.

47. Id.

48. See Minn. Pub. Health Dept. Regs. 367(e)(2), (5) (1974).

49. Philip C. Kissam, Ronald M. Johnson, "State HMO Laws and the Theory of Limited Reformmongering," Kansas Law Review 25(1976):21, 53.

50. Cal. Health & Safety Code §1367(f).

51. See N.J. Stat. Ann. §26-2J-11(a).

52. P.L. 93-406.

53. Id. §4(b)(3).

54. U.S. Department of Labor Press Release 78-188, March 10, 1978.

55. 442 F. Supp. 695(1977).

56. Id.

57. Id., 704.

58. 425 F. Supp. 1294 (1977).

59. 15U.S.C. §§1–7.

60. 423U.S.886 (1975).

61. Lawrence Sullivan, Antitrust, Chapter 3, "Horizontal Restraints on Trade," 186–189 (St. Paul: West Publishing, 1977).

62. Id., pp. 196–197.

63. Ward Kallstrom, "Health Care Cost Control by Third Party Payors: Fee Schedules and the Sherman Act," paper presented at the conference, "The Antitrust Laws nd the Health Services Industry," Washington, D.C., December 19–20, 1977.

64. Supra at n. 6.1, pp. 30–35.

65. Newsletter of the American Council of Otolarynogology, Vol. 9, No. 6, December 1977.

66. Supra at n. 63.

67. 15 U.S.C. §§1011–1015.

68. See McIlhinney v. American Title Insurance Co. 418 F. Supp. 364 (1977).

69. 424 F. Supp. 657 (1976).

70. 415 F. Supp. 343 (1976), U.S. Sup. Ct. 77-952.

71. U.S. Supreme Court 77-240, June 29, 1978.

Issues for the Future

Richard H. Egdahl, Diana Chapman Walsh,
and Joanna Lion

The defeat of the administration's hospital cost containment legislation by private sector advocates of "voluntary controls,"[1] coupled with the general message against government spending embodied in Proposition 13, might seem to herald the demise of the regulatory forces aligned against health care costs and an opportunity for providers to return to business as usual. If health care providers can effectively quell rising costs through voluntary efforts, then so much the better. But if they cannot? Then the predictable long-range consequence will be progressively more stringent regulation, perhaps ultimately culminating in nationalization of the health industry. Can voluntary controls succeed? If they amount to piecemeal efforts, the chances appear to be slim. The challenge will be to find systematic and sustained methods of controlling health care costs, while preserving the good features of the nation's pluralistic health care system.

The speculative discussion in this chapter begins with several assumptions.

1. Health care costs will continue to rise faster than the rate of increase in the gross national product. Fragmentary efforts to modulate costs will be frustrated by the inflationary imperative of health care delivery constantly changing to accommodate technological innovation and the growing demand for care which accompanies the national fascination with health, an aging population, a leisure society, and other ingrained social forces.

2. Pressures will build within the government, business, and labor for effective control of health care costs.

3. The unstructured, fee-for-service, cost-reimbursement system will be unable to respond effectively to these pressures.

4. Unless working models of alternatives to the unstructured system are operating in a few geographical areas and competing successfully on the basis of consumer preference and price, the pressure for cost control will inevitably lead to greater and more restrictive regulation.

Given these assumptions, the measure that seems to offer the best potential for control of all health care costs incurred by a given individual is a system of prepayment within a fixed budget. Such a system promotes tacit rationing which does not jeopardize essential health services because it merely takes up some of the considerable slack now existing in the system in the form of untested new technology, unproven and overlapping diagnostic and treatment procedures, and unchecked demand for optional but unessential health care services. A prepaid plan is a vehicle to organize the delivery of health care, effect rationing of nonessential services, introduce management efficiencies, and provide the leverage to hold health care costs in line with the general economy.

There is only one alternative to promoting competition or strengthening regulation: we could decide not to worry so much about costs. Uwe Reinhardt, an economist at Princeton University, suggests provocatively that health care costs may be a false problem.[2] Since Americans spend so much of their discretionary income on things that cause them harm, he argues, why not spend 12, 15, or 20 percent of our gross national product on health, instead of almost 9 percent now? Health care is, after all, a relatively benign indulgence that incidentally provides rewarding employment for some five million Americans.[3] On the editorial pages of the *Wall Street Journal*, Peter Drucker recently took a parallel tack.[4] He questioned whether the American public really cares about health care costs, and cited several public opinion polls that seem to indicate otherwise.

But if our assumptions *are* correct and granting our conclusion that prepayment is the only effective cost containment strategy short of massive regulation, we predict that corporations will continue searching for ways to contain their health care costs and will give serious consideration to sponsoring HMOs. In so doing, they will develop informal yardsticks to use as a basis for corporate assessment of the HMO option, and these, in turn, could profoundly alter the financing and delivery of health care in a kind of chain reaction of incremental corporate decisions. The sheer magnitude of the large corporations—the numbers of employees and their dependents and the levels of investment at stake—makes this impact almost automatic, whatever direction it may take.

Many issues for the future emerge from our series of assumptions; three stand out:

- For industry, the issue will be what yardsticks to use in assessing HMO sponsorship, what level of investment is warranted, and what kinds of expectations are reasonable.
- For HMOs, the issue for the future will be how to establish useful data bases and credible track records.
- For national health policy, the issue will be how to define and allocate whatever "savings" may be achieved through promoting HMOs.

The Issue for Industry: Setting Realistic Expectations and Goals

First, it is critical that corporations make long-range projections of their health benefit costs and try to implement procedures that will slow the rate of increase. Shorter term savings are an important but secondary goal, since they often occur on a one-time basis. In nearly every situation, effective prepaid health plans provide an opportunity to slow the rate of cost escalation. Short-term savings will depend on such specific circumstances as whether the existing package includes first dollar coverage, how rich the benefit package is, and what opportunities exist for the corporation to build particular innovations into the HMOs. Examples of the latter are providing in-house ancillary services; contracting with different hospitals for different types and levels of services and selecting them by their case mixes; arranging hospital discounts; and developing hybrid HMOs, such as modified open panels with careful screening of physicians, and other variations described in chapter 3.

If the goal of cost control is approached with realistic expectations and a willingness to innovate, industry's interests will best be served by efforts to stimulate, support, and sponsor prepaid health plans of both the salaried group and the fee-for-service variety. Society's interests will be served as well if consumers can be given an opportunity to make informed choices among health care plans. Corporate executives have traditionally been chary of interfering with the medical profession's expressed interests.[5] With the growing realization that more medical care is not necessarily better care, this automatic diffidence is slowly yielding to a more critical view. As industry assesses HMO development, a prime purpose should be to join providers in managing a health care delivery system that has the potential to maintain quality, control costs, and evaluate the products delivered.

The Issue for HMOs: Amassing Useful Data and Establishing Credible Records

Evidence is badly needed to demonstrate that various types of HMOs in diverse settings and stages of development are effective in containing costs. Anecdotal experience abounds, but it is not enough. The solid results recorded by well-established prepaid plans are suggestive but not conclusive for the general case. The fact remains that reliable measures must be found with which to assess the relative performance of various types of salaried group, fee-for-service, and direct capitation HMOs.

One measure of performance is the quality of health care; and there is no evidence that quality suffers in an HMO. The intensity of peer review carried out by most HMOs should actually help assure uniform standards of care. Ellwood calls on HMOs to monitor their own quality, lest their detractors charge that they are controlling costs at their patients' expense.[6] Consumer choice in a functioning market—the ultimate goal of the HMO movement—is a built-in safeguard for quality.

Another criterion of performance is the cost of delivering health care services in a range of settings. Although cost comparisons are problematic because different benefit packages seldom match exactly, hospital days per 1,000 enrollees is frequently used as a proxy measure of costs. Hospital days are expensive and therefore of major interest; also, they are relatively easier to count than other medical encounters.

The recent HMO census survey[7] illustrates the difficulty of using this statistic as a performance measure. The census covered 165 currently functioning prepaid plans, only eleven of which did not report at all. Twenty-eight more could not report on the number of hospital days per 1,000 enrollees. For the 126 plans reporting this statistic, the mean and median were close to 500 days per 1,000 population (519 and 488, respectively), but the *range* was extensive—from 124 to 1,462 days. At the low end was a plan serving college students, whereas one-quarter of the members of the plan at the high end were Medicare patients. The point is obvious: the population must be standardized for at least age (and sex because of maternity days) before days per 1,000 can be used as a meaningful comparative measure.

Studies which have standardized for age and sex, such as those Luft recently reviewed,[8] demonstrate the savings potential of the prepaid group practice HMOs. Less is known about fee-for-service HMOs, and researchers have tended to seize on the only available data, however outdated, and from them to impugn the potential of recent, quite different, generations of fee-for-service HMOs. Research is needed to identify age- and sex-standardized utilization in these newer plans and to isolate the causes of variation. What are the effects of the different utilization control programs? Does a preadmission certification program reduce the admission rate generally, or does it primarily affect certain diagnoses? What happens to those patients who are no longer admitted? Are their admissions simply postponed, or are they treated on an outpatient basis? Does a concurrent review program reduce the length of stay? If so, does this reduction occur at the beginning by reducing the preoperative length of stay, or at the end? What are the effects of different levels of risk? Do the physicians change their behavior as the percent of fees withheld increases? How does the percent of a physician's practice which is in the HMO influence his behavior? When it is a small part of his practice, with only a minor impact on his income, does he treat his HMO patients differently, perhaps in a more cost conscious manner from the remainder of his practice? At what percent does the HMO become a consequential portion of the physician's practice? What effect does reaching this level have on his practice pattern, both for his HMO patients and for his other patients?

Specific data are required to answer these kinds of questions, including accurate coding of diagnoses and treatment, as well as basic patient information covering such variables as age, previous medical history, concurrent outpatient treatment, and the like. Another requirement is specific demographic data about enrollees. For example, if only a small proportion of enrollees are children, a low tonsillectomy rate compared to that of a traditionally insured group means little.

To develop track records based on number of hospital days per 1,000 enrollees, fee-for-service HMOs should collect sufficient data to identify what components of hospitalization are being reduced and where trade-offs are being made for other types of care. *Ideally*, this data should include:

> primary discharge diagnosis;
>
> secondary diagnoses;
>
> all procedures;
>
> total length of stay;
>
> length of stay prior to primary procedure;
>
> outpatient care (including outpatient surgery, physician encounters, and paramedical encounters);
>
> demographic data about inpatient populations;
>
> demographic data about subscriber population.

We emphasize "ideally" because, as corporate executives who deal with employee health benefits know well, traditional health insurance carriers— whether Blue Cross or commercial companies—tend to keep claims-oriented data systems. Such a system usually permits verification only that the employee is covered under a family contract rather than as an individual and the level of benefits purchased. Data such as the number, age, and sex of dependents are generally outside the scope of a claims-oriented system, and the diagnostic and procedural codes used are usually quite rough.

Some fee-for-service HMOs also have claims-oriented data systems. As a matter of public policy, it is essential that an additional investment be made to enable at least a few of these newer types of prepaid health plan to collect meaningful data and establish records that can be studied and, where warranted, emulated.

The Broader Policy Issue: Who Ought to Realize the Savings?

The third issue for the future concerns national health policy; specifically, what are the savings and who should benefit from them? HMOs are believed to stimulate competition in health care through economic incentives. Because these incentives derive from the savings that HMOs can achieve, it is important to ask what altered behavior the savings ought to reward or inspire. The HMO savings are a little like the proverb of the blind men and the elephant. The picture changes completely with shifts in the vantage point.

Physicians are the chief decision makers in the health care system. Because they commit most expenditures for medical care, the incentives governing their choices are obviously important. No HMO can succeed without physician leadership—least of all fee-for-service HMOs, which involve large numbers of physicians in a comparatively loose management structure. To portray physicians' incentives as purely economic is an oversimplification; nevertheless, on the health care balance sheet physicians have much at stake. Physician fees are increasingly under attack and the medical profession is concerned that the country will drift into a nationalized health system. Fee-for-service HMOs usually spring up in response to the immediate threat of salaried group plans and are fortified by more remote concerns about the future of private practice. Participation in fee-for-service HMOs requires considerable change on the part of physicians. Most will not become involved unless they see participation as an accommodation to practical necessity, yielding a reasonable return on a major investment of effort. The investigations by the Massachusetts Division of Insurance into the application of the Bay State Health Care Foundation are described in appendix II. The consumer group opposing that plan has questioned the motives of its organizing physicians. But without some faith that HMO savings will help protect their incomes, physicians seem unlikely to exert the effort required to control costs. The physician's feel of the HMO savings elephant encourages him to conclude that it is a creature which can preserve the level of his fees.

Hospitals gain the least in the HMO calculus. Although labor-intensive, hospitals have high fixed costs. To survive they must keep their unit costs down and their volumes up. The HMO's savings reflect reduced hospitalization at a time when regulatory agencies are becoming less tolerant of slack in hospital occupancy rates and are better able, through health planning and certificate-of-need programs, to enforce rigorous standards of efficiency. Complicating this issue is the fact that the reins on hospitals will be tightened at the expense of jobs—in a service industry where minorities are heavily represented. In most urban areas there are too many hospital beds.[9,10] The forward-looking administrators and trustees of hospitals see the inevitability of major change in the health care system over the next ten years. They ask themselves whether their institutions will survive the transition, and conclude that to do so they must act now to carve out a future niche. For most this means shrinking and shifting their priorities. A way to offset the inevitable loss of revenue will be to increase the hospital's relative share of the market of available patients. Some hospitals may seek to do this by sponsoring an HMO either alone or together with partners. This sets up a Darwinian dynamic where the fit survive by taking from the weak.

Meanwhile, hospitals that are struggling may have a legitimate short-term claim on some portion of HMO savings won at their expense to amortize the costs associated with relocating employees, consolidating units, and phasing out unneeded services. The various interests represented in the hospital sector will try hard to grab hold of at least a piece of the elephant and find there some needed help.

Industry pays an annual health insurance bill of some $30 billion and feels acutely the pinch of steadily rising costs. Chapter 2 described how several large corporations are now assessing the feasibility of sponsoring HMOs. As noted in chapter 3, R. J. Reynolds Corporation has already taken the step by creating the Winston-Salem Health Care Plan for its employees. Reynolds had several reasons for starting this HMO, but the "final push" came from the need to moderate the increase in the company's medical premium expenses— amounting to a 20 percent rise each year since 1970.[11] A shortage of practicing physicians in Winston-Salem provided Reynolds with unusually fertile ground for HMO development. Other companies with comparable cost problems may face medical community hostility, which Reynolds was spared. But if they become convinced that sponsorship of HMOs will enable them to contain their health care costs without sacrificing quality, some corporations may find ways to neutralize provider opposition. If industry sees a way to offer health services of equal quality at substantially lower cost, the imperative of the bottom line may well prevail.

Competing claims on HMO savings are an implicit part of the interest expressed in various sectors—management, labor, hospitals, physicians, insurance carriers, and others—in the HMO movement. So far, the issue of who should share in the savings realized by HMOs has received little overt attention. But it is now time to address the matter. Otherwise, HMO savings could easily be balkanized before they are even fully documented. If each interested sector expects to reap the total potential benefit, unrealistically high expectations will quickly yield to disillusionment, and the HMO movement will lose its diverse constituency and much of its momentum. Given the assumptions enumerated at the beginning of this chapter, the ensuing dissipation of support would be an undesirable outcome, since society needs the aggregate control of costs that HMOs seem capable of providing. Competition is a new concept for the health care system and many questions remain. But it is time to begin asking them systematically; competition should have a true test.

NOTES

1. "Hospital Cost Cap Bill Deflated by House Commerce Committee," *Washington Report on Medicine and Health 32* (30) (Washington, D.C.: McGraw-Hill, July 24, 1978), p. 2.

2. Uwe E. Reinhardt, "Four Perspectives—Where Will We Be in Five Years?" *Controlling Health Care Costs: A National Leadership Conference* (Washington, D.C.: Government Research Corporation, 1978), pp. 11–15.

3. U.S. Department of Health, Education, and Welfare: *Health—United States—1976–1977* (Washington, D.C.: DHEW Publication No. (HRA) 77-1232. National Center for Health Statistics and National Center for Health Services Research, 1978).

4. Peter F. Drucker, "The Future Shape of Health Care," *Wall Street Journal*, Wednesday, July 19, 1978, p. 12.

5. Diana Chapman Walsh and Richard H. Egdahl, *Payer, Provider, Consumer: Industry Confronts Health Care Costs*, Springer Series on Industry and Health Care, No. 1 (New York: Springer-Verlag, 1977).

6. Paul M. Ellwood, Jr., "The Importance of the Market," *Journal of Health Politics, Policy and Law 2*(4) (Winter, 1978): 447–453.

7. Group Health Association of America, *National HMO Census Survey—1977* (Washington, D.C.: Group Health Association of America, 1978).

8. Harold S. Luft, "How Do Health Maintenance Organizations Achieve Their Savings?" *New England Journal of Medicine 298* (June 15, 1978): 1336–1343.

9. Walter McClure, "Reducing Excess Hospital Capacity," (Washington, D.C.: prepared by InterStudy for the Bureau of Health Planning and Development, Department of Health, Education, and Welfare, contract no. HRA-230-76-0086, October 15, 1976.)

10. Institute of Medicine, *Controlling the Supply of Hospital Beds* (Washington, D.C.: National Academy of Sciences, 0-309-02610-5, October, 1976).

11. Bynum E. Tudor, "A New Corporate Prepaid Group Health Plan," in Richard H. Egdahl, ed., *Background Papers on Industry's Changing Role in Health Care Delivery*, Springer Series on Industry and Health Care, No. 3 (New York: Springer-Verlag, 1977).

Appendix I

A National Call to Action: Secretary Califano's HMO Conference

Anthony J. Mahler

> *. . . we have asked you here today to call upon the great institution-building skill of American business and labor, and to enlist that skill in coping with the problem of soaring health costs—in your interest and in the nation's.*
>
> Secretary Califano
> (luncheon address)

Secretary Califano's call to action at the HMO conference was a plea from the government to the private sector to help make the nation's health care system work efficiently and effectively. The meeting was not intended as a how-to session; as Califano cautioned, "we offer no prescriptions." Rather, the conference was devoted to communicating a simple theme: HMOs offer a good system of controlled health care, one that both management and labor can and should support. This message was dramatized by reporting the experience of several unions and companies in developing HMOs.

The conference was divided into four segments. The first explored the concept of HMOs and what they can offer industry and labor. The second segment presented three cases of industry- or labor-sponsored HMOs, noting particular obstacles and how these were overcome. The third segment was devoted to the federal commitment to the HMO concept, with a luncheon address by Secretary Califano and speeches by three key Congressional representatives who support HMOs. In the final segment, a panel focused on what the Department of Health, Education, and Welfare can do to help, given that HMO development must be primarily a private-sector activity.

More than 1,300 participants, including representatives of some 320 large corporations, were welcomed by HEW Under Secretary Hale Champion, who sketched the current picture of health care costs and the role of HMOs in changing this picture. Health care costs now consume some 12 percent of all tax dollars, and their rate of inflation is two and one-half times that of the general economy. The only part of the system which has managed to buck this inflationary spiral has been the HMO. Its emphasis on quality and continuity of care, coupled with the ability to practice prevention and maintenance, is impressive. Equally impressive is the financial performance of HMOs, which have reduced hospitalization for their enrollees by 30 to 60 percent. Most of the savings generated by this reduction have been returned to the purchaser of HMO services: total costs per enrollee range from 10 to 40 percent less for groups, and around 20 percent less for Medicaid recipients. But the HMO option is still not widely available. There are only about 170 HMOs, with 6.5 million members, nationwide.

The first of the two keynote speeches was given by George Meany, President of the AFL-CIO. He opened his presentation by affirming the strong support of both labor and management for the HMO movement, as represented by the consensus position paper issued by the informal, private Labor-Management Group, which he co-chaired. Meany then presented organized labor's perspective on the HMO movement. Labor is appalled by the ever-increasing portion of workers' total compensation which must be devoted to health insurance, retarding the growth of wages and other fringe benefits. The problem, as Meany sees it, is the insatiable appetite of doctors and hospitals for more money, abetted by the fee-for-service payment system. The best remedy for this problem is the creation of nonprofit prepaid group practices. Meany does not support HMOs in all forms, and he particularly opposes those which are either for profit or based on fee-for-service reimbursement. In his view, the virtue of prepaid group practices is that they benefit patients, not doctors.

The AFL-CIO has sponsored or spearheaded many prepaid group practices and will continue to do so for two reasons. First, the prepaid group practice is the best buy for the dollar, providing the greatest benefit in the least costly fashion. Second, it delivers high-quality care, largely through careful screening of doctors who are hired, tight peer review, use of shared medical records, and emphasis on prevention and lifetime monitoring.

Meany concluded by noting that labor and management share the common goal of providing high-quality care at a low cost to workers and their families. Together, the two sectors can exert power as the buyers of health care services. HMOs are one of several mechanisms to achieve this goal. Through collective bargaining, labor and management can and should have a say in the health care system.

The other keynoter was Charles Pilliod, Chairman of the Board of Goodyear Tire and Rubber Company, who described a broader vision of the private-sector possibilities for prepaid health plans. He would like to see the growth of all forms—nonprofit and for profit—including prepaid group practices, IPAs, industrial hybrids, and others which do not yet exist. The key to system reform is the restructuring of incentives for both providers and consumers. The providers need incentives to practice in a cost-effective manner within a competitive system. The consumers, who surveys show are generally satisfied with the medical care they receive, need incentives to seek lower cost medical care, either through organized systems or through cost-conscious selection of providers. All parties must be involved if the goals of increased productivity and reduced waste are to be reached.

Pilliod also stressed the importance of finding a private-sector solution to the problem of health care costs. Mandatory cost controls will not be effective and will, in fact, have negative consequences. Voluntary controls, particularly through the market mechanism, are the preferred solution. HMOs are a part of this solution, but not the total answer. They will grow too slowly, owing in large part to the lack of qualified and experienced administrators. But they do provide the consumer with an alternative to the current system, and the consumer is the heart of an operating market.

Finally, Pilliod raised two concerns in the broader perspective of providing health care to the nation. First, the anticipated national health insurance proposal must include a major role for competing delivery systems, or else such systems will not survive. Second, the main concern of national health policy is to provide care to all who need it. The biggest problem now is the fact that some Americans do not receive care; formation of HMOs will not solve this problem.

HMOs and the Competitive Market

The first panel covered some of the basic issues in HMO development. John Boardman, Executive Vice President of Kaiser-Permanente Advisory Services, traced the development of the present system from early in the century, when nearly all medical services were purchased directly by the consumer, to the current system, in which third-party payers account for the bulk of reimbursement to health care providers. The fact that out-of-pocket costs now account for only 32 percent of total costs, and that many services are provided at no direct cost, has made price ineffectual as a regulator of health care supply and demand.

Boardman stated that labor, management, and government are now struggling to regain control over health care costs. One approach has been to tinker with the present system. However, tinkering may mask the need for structural change in the health care system. The development of HMOs represents an attempt to deal with some of the structural problems. The HMO is an organized system of care which guarantees delivery of needed services to a voluntarily enrolled population for a pre-established fee, as opposed to the prevailing health insurance system. All the various models of HMOs have potential as remedies, and labor and management should consider involvement ranging from sponsorship to providing the HMO alternative to their workers.

Alain Enthoven, Professor of Public and Private Management at Stanford University, gave an economist's view of HMOs. He started by addressing the question of whether HMOs save money and, if so, why. The answer he gave is that they do, by creating incentives to lower hospital utilization. The need to live within a fixed budget provides an incentive for efficiency which is absent, or even negative, in the traditional system. Enthoven highlighted the importance of changing incentives by drawing a parallel with the performance one would expect under a fixed-cost contract versus a cost-plus contract. He also pointed out that because HMOs compete directly for members, further incentives are created to avoid underservice while seeking to minimize costs. Of course, as in industry, some HMOs are more efficient than others. But the evidence indicates that the tougher the competition, the greater the savings achieved by the HMO. As an example, he noted that Hawaii has two HMOs which compete with each other, as well as with the traditional insurers, and these prepaid plans have achieved significant reductions in hospital utilization.

HMOs do not save money by underserving their members, according to Enthoven, who pointed out that there is no documentation of underservice. Furthermore, the increasing market penetration of HMOs tends to indicate that consumers do not perceive the prepaid plan as an underutilizer. Finally, HMOs have long served such highly educated groups as university faculties—groups which are quick to express their dissatisfaction. The continued success of HMOs in enrolling and serving such groups indicates that these enrollees are satisfied that they are receiving high-quality care.

Why, then, aren't there more HMOs serving larger numbers of people? Enthoven believes they have not had a fair chance to compete for several reasons. First, the traditional system has worked against them. While this is changing, as evidenced by the recent American Medical Association Cost Control Commission Report, there are still cases of hospitals denying HMO physicians staff privileges and thus preventing HMO expansion.

A second reason is that federal law has been biased against HMOs. The original HMO Act did as much to discourage their development by imposing unreasonable standards as it did to encourage them through grants and loans. Tax law also discourages competition by treating all employer contributions to health insurance premiums as nontaxable income to employees, and thus encouraging employees to seek comprehensive insurance which is fully paid for, thereby further insulating them from the cost consequences of their decisions. This leads to the third reason HMOs have not had a fair chance to compete: the lack of incentives for people to join such alternative systems. While particularly acute for Medicaid and Medicare recipients, this problem also figures in cases where employee health insurance is mostly or completely paid by the employer.

Beyond the obstacles to fair competition, Enthoven observed that the major reason why HMOs are not more prevalent is that they do not spring up by themselves. Effective local efforts are required in the development, marketing, and financing of HMOs. Corporations can realize significant cost savings by undertaking such activities to sponsor HMOs in their communities. The alternative strategies, such as modifying existing benefit packages or relying on government regulation to control costs, hold little prospect for success.

The next speaker, Kenneth Bannon, Vice President of the United Auto Workers and President of Metro Health Plan in Detroit, presented the labor view on HMOs. Like Meany, he expressed strong support for nonprofit prepaid group practices. The UAW encourages its local officials to become involved in HMO development and has established four such plans. Based on this experience, Bannon identified five major obstacles to the successful marketing of a prepaid group practice. First, UAW members already have comprehensive benefits, and thus the prepaid group practice has little to offer them on this score. Second, union members and their spouses tend to be loyal to the physicians with whom they have established relationships. Third, because the workers are unfamiliar with HMOs, they are reluctant to join such an unknown entity. Fourth, they may have heard more bad than good reports of prepaid group practices. Stories often circulate that there is a long waiting period for appointments, the emergency room is like a zoo, and members cannot have their own doctors. Finally, there is often an additional premium payment to be made, especially for new plans.

The UAW stands ready to help start prepaid group practices and will work to encourage its members to join them. Bannon emphasized the importance of involving the local union early in the development process in order to gain labor support for the plan. Furthermore, he suggested that labor unions and companies should devote some time and effort to pre-enrollment education. Bannon also noted that assuring prospective enrollees that they will have "their own doctor" would influence enrollment significantly.

The business view on HMOs was provided by Stanley King, Assistant Vice President for Personnel, American Telephone and Telegraph. King stated that business has two major concerns with HMO development: cost and benefit. The cost of health care for business is rising at a greater rate than total personnel costs and is an increasingly important part of the cost of doing business. But, King cautioned, business should not expect a quick fix from the HMO movement. The plans themselves may not be cheaper unless care is taken to insure that the savings realized from reduced hospitalization are not eaten up by increased ambulatory benefits.

Assuming, however, that an HMO is operating efficiently, the cost savings will still be negligible for the corporate sponsor unless a large number of employees is willing to join and remain in the plan. Only 10 percent of eligible AT&T employees have elected to enroll in an HMO—only 6 percent, excluding California and Minnesota. Any savings may be offset by the increased administrative costs associated with having small numbers of employees enrolled in several plans across the country. Furthermore, many struggling HMOs require subsidies in order to continue to survive.

King speculated that employees probably do not choose between plans on the basis of cost but rather on the basis of coverage. This is particularly true when the employer pays the full premium, since the employee is unlikely to choose a plan simply to save the employer money. Therefore, the HMO has to deliver the goods if it expects to attract and hold a large membership.

The second major concern for business is the benefits that HMOs provide their members. As responsible employers, companies want to provide their employees with high-quality health care. Thus, a company should offer an HMO as one of several choices, even if there are no cost savings, as long as the HMO is delivering a good product. The company may realize an indirect saving, in terms of reduced disability or sick days.

The last speaker on this panel was Dr. Ernest Saward, Professor of Medicine at the University of Rochester, who spoke on the reality of physician participation in HMOs. Saward stated that, as systems of medical care delivery, HMOs cannot work without the active commitment of their physicians. Organized medicine has not always been favorable to these kinds of plans. But today the situation has changed. Physicians are not only available but eager to join HMOs. Only a minority of new doctors entering practice choose to go into solo practice; the majority opt for partnerships, single-specialty groups, or multispecialty groups.

In particular, Saward noted, the prepaid group practices are attractive to physicians. They offer ready access to qualified peers, provide the required technology, and make use of shared medical records. Also, prepaid group practices encourage physicians to practice appropriate medicine. There is no incentive to use hospital rather than ambulatory care; the emphasis on preventive medicine and continuity of care allows physicians to assume responsibility for the total health of their patients, and the team practice approach facilitates efficient use of ancillary personnel. In fact, the reduced hospitalization in prepaid group practices is caused not so much by changed incentives as it is by appropriate use and planning of resources. Finally, joining a prepaid group practice eliminates the problems of setting up and running a solo practice.

Dr. Saward closed with a few thoughts on the appropriate role in HMO development for employers and unions, which he thinks should exert a strong, but seldom a controlling, influence. They must take a positive stance and underscore the advantages of HMOs, since a passive role will not do the job. On the other hand, employers and unions must not force enrollment by offering HMOs as the only available plan. Multiple choice, with its emphasis on voluntarily enrolled populations, is necessary for HMO success.

To summarize, this first panel laid the groundwork for the rest of the conference. It covered the genesis of the current problem of health care costs, the role of the HMO in addressing the problem, and the evidence on the performance of HMOs. The basic attitudes of business, labor, and medicine toward HMOs were clearly expressed.

Studies of Corporate and Labor Involvement

The second segment of the conference, consisting of a panel moderated by Dr. Paul Ellwood, President of InterStudy, focused on the experiences of two companies and one labor union in sponsoring or acting as catalyst for HMOs. While these cases were not necessarily presented as models, the obstacles faced by the three organizations are typical of those hindering any such effort. The lessons that were learned may be helpful to others who intend to take an active role in HMO development.

Paul Parker, Executive Vice President of General Mills, spoke on the role that industry played in HMO development in Minneapolis. In 1971–72, General Mills sought alternatives to its standard approach to corporate philanthropy, and decided to concentrate on managing and organizing public service activities rather than on writing checks. At about that time, Dr. Leon Warshaw of the Equitable Life Assurance Society of America proposed that General Mills study the potential for HMOs in Minneapolis.

However, General Mills, deciding it was more interested in action than study, organized the Twin City Health Care Development Project, sponsored by eleven companies and eight insurers. The goal of the Project was to develop several HMOs in Minneapolis. While all of the members did not move at an equal pace, the goal was eventually achieved—there are now eight HMOs in the city. During the years of development, project members discovered that the ability of a company to move quickly is related to the level of involvement of corporate officers. General Mills had involved corporate officers from the start of the project, while some other companies had involved only their personnel departments. There were also conflicts with the insurance companies over the issue of control. The insurers envisioned the HMOs as part of their business, while the companies wanted them to operate as independent entities.

Parker noted that three lessons were learned from the experience. First, the providers and the community at large should be involved in the process from the beginning. In the Twin City Project, they were only brought in at a late date, a factor which probably slowed the development effort. Second, it is important to work for a pluralistic system, since this kind of competition breeds survivors. The HMOs in Minneapolis compete not only with traditional insurance but with each other. While perhaps not all of them will make it, those which do will be strong organizations. Third, crusading should be avoided. Good educational efforts, such as working with small groups on company time, are important to success, but it is equally critical not to oversell. HMOs must be presented as an alternative system, not a better system.

What are the results? General Mills now has 60 percent of its Minneapolis employees enrolled in HMOs (although only 5 percent of those employed elsewhere belong to such a plan). The advantages for General Mills have been a boost in morale among its work force, provision of additional benefits at an equal or lower cost, and a significant reduction in employee hospitalization. The unadjusted figures are 800 days per 1,000 for employees in the traditional plan versus 375 days per 1,000 for those enrolled in HMOs. The major unanswered question is whether or not the HMOs are leading to a healthier work force.

Dr. Ellwood noted that Minneapolis exemplified another characteristic of HMO development—the fact that they seem to cluster. The 170 HMOs in the country tend to be concentrated in a few areas. In fact, about four-fifths of all standard metropolitan statistical areas do not yet have operating HMOs. The hopeful side of this phenomenon is that development of one HMO in an area may serve as the catalyst for starting others; that is, it may have a multiplier effect.

The story of a union-sponsored HMO was presented by Edwin Brown, Secretary-Treasurer of the Rhode Island AFL-CIO. In 1966 the Rhode Island council began to consider the need to change the health care delivery system. To assist in this effort, the Group Health Association of America sent Thomas Ludwig to Rhode Island to perform an HMO feasibility study. Prompted by Ludwig's positive recommendation, member unions were asked to commit themselves to the development of a prepaid group practice. They did so, providing some $300,000 in seed money.

There were a number of difficulties to overcome during the development phase. First, special state legislation was required to exempt the plan from insurance laws. Second, the union sought, but did not obtain, employer support for the planning and development of the HMO. The largest obstacle was the strong opposition of organized medicine to the union plan. As a result of this opposition, participating physicians were denied staff privileges at all of the area hospitals. This problem was finally solved by gaining the support of the bishop, who ordered the Catholic hospital in his diocese to cooperate, thereby allowing the plan to become operational. Subsequent management problems were overcome by signing a management contract with the Prudential Insurance Company of America. The plan became the first federally qualified HMO on October 30, 1975.

Dr. Charles Ryan, Corporate Medical Director of the Sun Company, presented the final case: an IPA on the verge of commencing operations. Its genesis can be traced back to the early 1970s, when the Sun Company started looking at the escalating costs of the traditional health care system. It appeared that most physicians felt trapped by the system, with its distorted incentives. The medical sector also expressed concern about the few physicians who did not practice good medicine, but felt powerless to do anything about them.

The passage of the HMO Act in 1973 turned the Sun Company's attention to the five prepaid group practices being developed in Philadelphia. Although corporate investigators liked the HMO concept, they felt that these plans would not adequately serve Sun Company employees, who live mostly to the south and west of Philadelphia. Therefore, they approached a major hospital in the area, which agreed to explore the possibility of an HMO tailored to the needs of the Delaware Valley population. After obtaining the approval of the corporate management, the Sun Company investigators formed an organization comprising nine other companies and three of the six local hospitals, which in turn hired a consultant to perform a feasibility study. Fifteen other companies in the area participated but did not contribute money to the organization.

The feasibility study concentrated on marketing potential and physician participation. The study found that 70 percent of the employees of the participating companies lived within three miles of one of the three hospitals. Penetration was estimated at 6 percent in the first year, 15 percent in the second, and 20 percent in the third, which would provide a sufficient base for a viable plan. The study also found that area physicians were strongly opposed to any prepaid group practice plan, but that 300 out of 650 would be willing to participate in an IPA. Therefore, it was decided to proceed with the development of an IPA plan based on the medical staffs of the three hospitals.

However, when the companies were again asked for funds, only four were willing to contribute. A new organization was formed and the board was expanded to include community representation. Subcommittees were created to plan the various parts of the HMO. The planning and development phase took two and one-half years to complete, in part because of insufficient funds. To resolve this problem, the plan sought and obtained federal funding. It was decided that the chairman of the board should be a provider in order to lessen the anxiety of area physicians. The plan opened to patients on April 1, 1978.

Dr. Ellwood summed up the experiences reported by the panel by listing some of the different sponsoring roles played by industry and unions in HMO development. Apart from outright ownership, industry and unions can provide leadership, find capital, make key personnel available to assist the HMO, provide strong support of the option, and make the idea legitimate in the community. Whatever the role assumed, he said, it is important that industry and unions become increasingly involved in the HMO movement.

The Call to Action

The major speech of the day was the luncheon address by HEW Secretary Joseph Califano. He called upon "the problem-solving genius of America's private sector" to focus on the problem of health care cost control. To illustrate the cost problem, he recited the experience of the Ford Motor Company. In 1965 Ford spent $68 million on health care, with an average of $350 for each active employee. By 1977 the figure had grown to $450 million, or $2,000 per employee; and Ford estimates that in 1979 these costs will reach $630 million, or $2,700 per employee. "And what is true for Ford is true for American business generally. In one year alone, from 1975 to 1976, spending for group health insurance skyrocketed by $5 billion—more than 20 percent—and the cost is still rising."

Secretary Califano summarized the reasons for this cost problem:

> . . . the very qualities that have made the American economy the envy of the world; the very qualities that are rightly cherished in most of the American marketplace—that encourage quality and wide distribution of services at a reasonable cost—are glaringly absent from the health economy; consumer choice is largely absent, incentives to keep costs low are absent, rational planning is scant, and competition is almost nonexistent.

HMOs represent one way to change this situation, and they offer three major advantages: quality, efficiency, and cost savings. On the third point, Secretary Califano noted that, with only 5 percent of its employees enrolled in HMOs, Ford estimates it saved $2 million over comparable traditional insurance costs in 1977. "If only 5 percent of the employees of the Fortune 500 had enrolled last year in HMOs, that modest enrollment would have saved up to $150 million—with no sacrifice in quality." Despite this potential, and despite the efforts of the federal government, HMO enrollment accounts for only 3 percent of the nation's population.

"So today I lay before you a challenge and an opportunity: We are asking you, as leaders and decision makers whose combined impact on the marketplace can be enormous, to encourage the spread of HMOs. We offer no prescriptions. We hold up no preconceived perfect model to be followed. We ask simply that you consider these alternatives, in your own self-interest." Secretary Califano urged the audience to support existing HMOs and those in the process of being developed, join community groups organized to launch new HMOs, assume leadership roles in developing HMOs, and "invest in competition and quality health care by lending corporate dollars and management talent to HMOs—realizing that your returns will be in dollars saved."

This should be a private-sector effort. "In fact, we are convinced that, when it comes to developing HMOs, anything government can do, you can do better." What government can do is help. For example, HEW has taken, or is taking, a number of steps to increase the effectiveness of its own effort. All HMO activities are now grouped under a single administrator, Howard Veit. The department is stepping up its technical assistance and monitoring activities; working to streamline procedures and reduce paperwork; exploring new concepts, such as HMO networks, to minimize the administrative burden to large corporations; and working with Congress to rewrite the HMO Act in order to increase its effectiveness. However, Secretary Califano emphasized that "whether HMOs become a widespread feature of our health care system depends far more upon what you do than what we do. We will be more cooperative; we will give maximum assistance. We intend this to be primarily the private sector's effort. And I need not tell you that this may be one of the last chances for American free enterprise to tackle the task."

HMOs will not provide an overnight solution to the problem. They are but one part of an overall effort to bring costs under control. "First of all, you can approach your purchase of health benefits as you would approach the purchase of steel or raw materials, with an eye to cost-effectiveness as well as quality." Analysis of utilization patterns may suggest some strategies, and it may be possible to renegotiate benefit packages to remove some of the perverse incentives. Stepped-up prevention programs could also yield impressive results. Finally, an active role in the health planning process can help discourage excess capacity in the health care system.

> So today we launch a hopeful new effort—an effort to bring to the nation's health care system the efficiency and vitality of America's private sector. Doing that is in the interest of business—for cost savings are the essence of good business. It is also in the interest of labor—for those dollars saved could mean higher take-home pay or other benefits. And it is in the interest of the nation—for tax dollars now spent on health care could be used for other public purposes—or for lower taxes. Our challenge, yours and mine, is to forge our self-interests into shared interests.

Secretary Califano was followed, in the third segment of the conference, by three major Congressional figures concerned with HMOs. The first was Congressman Paul Rogers, Chairman of the House Subcommittee on Public Health and the Environment, who traced the troubled history of the HMO Act and its implementation:

> One of the biggest challenges faced by the House health subcommittee since I have been chairman was the development of an HMO bill which was acceptable to a sufficient number of subcommittee members to insure its passage. HMOs represented—to many—a radical departure from the health care delivery system we were so familiar with and, as such, generated immense controversy.

However many compromises and modifications required to create a bill suc-
ceeded, "and for all of its problems, the HMO Act of 1973 represented a
commitment by government to insuring the development of an alternative
system of health care, one that paid attention to both quality and costs while
strongly emphasizing prevention and health education."

"We soon learned that the 1973 legislation, instead of fostering competition, was almost anticompetitive in nature. We in the Congress had asked too
much of HMOs. We asked that they deliver, as basic benefits, health services for
which most third-party payers don't provide reimbursement." Many of these
well-intentioned requirements were modified by the 1976 amendments.

There was another serious problem for the HMO program:

> It is common knowledge that the previous administration backed
> away from its vigorous pro-HMO stance soon after enactment of
> the 1973 legislation. A woefully understaffed HMO office was
> downgraded. Incredible delays in writing regulations ensued be-
> cause of unresolved policy issues. No guidelines were issued with
> respect to expansion requests or conditions which HMOs must
> meet in order to become federally qualified.

Fortunately, the Carter administration has renewed the commitment to
the program, and the Congress stands willing to help however it can.

> Ultimately, management and labor—the people in this room—will
> have to decide whether HMOs are truly a national movement in-
> volving national enterprise or simply a noble experiment. For
> HMOs to succeed, they will need the management talent, marketing
> expertise, the private capital, and the commitment that only you
> can provide. I hope your decision will be to make HMOs into a
> broad-based national movement, and look forward to working with
> you in attaining that goal.

Senator Edward Kennedy, Chairman of the Senate Subcommittee on
Health and Scientific Research, agreed that the HMO climate has changed
dramatically since 1972. "A new consensus is emerging on the validity and
importance of the HMO concept. The new administration has made a firm
commitment to improve the management and funding of the program. We in
Congress will help them to honor that commitment in every way we can. . . ."
Among other things, the new HMO bill "proposes to end the experimental
status of the HMO program and make it a full-fledged, long-term federal effort."
This and other recent developments confirm Kennedy's long-held belief that
"HMOs are an essential element in our strategy for making the American health
care system more humane, effective, and efficient. . . ."

> There is an appropriate role for large corporations and labor
> unions in promoting the growth and development of HMOs. Your
> organization and the American people generally would benefit
> greatly from the wide availability of HMOs, and there is much you
> can do to make the HMO movement stronger. Secretary Califano

has already pointed to a number of possible actions, and I fully support most of these suggestions.

Senator Kennedy cited increased educational activities for employees, financial assistance for developing HMOs, and provision of managerial talent and financial expertise as appropriate actions.

"At the same time, however, I have profound reservations about any direct involvement of your firms in starting and running your own HMOs, especially if they are to be run for profit. Even without the profit incentive, your organizations stand to benefit substantially from the saving to be realized if large numbers of your employees use prepaid plans." The danger of the profit motive is that the health care providers may then have divided loyalties, whereas they "should be loyal only to their own patients."

The last speaker on this panel was Senator Richard Schweiker, Ranking Minority Member of the Senate Subcommittee on Health and Scientific Research. He began by expressing strong bipartisan support for the HMO effort:

Why do I, a Republican, support this initiative? Because I see HMOs as a step away from government regulation. HMOs stimulate competition in health care—competition with the fee-for-service system and competition with other HMOs. Where there is competition, there can be less regulation. HMOs can avoid regulation because they contain internal cost and quality incentives. . . . Competition, positive incentives, and a proven record—all are sound Republican principles.

In order to improve the HMO program, Senator Schweiker said, he has recently introduced a bill to amend the HMO Act. Among the more significant provisions are authorization for a management training program, which will emphasize field experience; increased funding, both for the program and for individual HMOs; and financial support for continuing development and operation of HMOs. The main theme of the legislation "is to change the HMO concept from a demonstration program to a permanent reform."

Senator Schweiker made one final point:

There's no reason that HMO development has to occur only within the federal rules and regulations. There are many variations of HMOs worth examining. Some forms are tried and true—they're the ones you can get federal money for starting. Others have yet to prove themselves. Still others have yet to be invented. If you can start an HMO without the federal government, more power to you! If you can develop new kinds of HMOs that deliver quality care at a reasonable community cost, do it! Washington has a lot to learn from the collective genius of the private sector. Let your imaginations and expertise go to work. This is your chance to show Washington how it's done. Don't pass it up!

The message of this third segment was clear: the federal government is committed to supporting the creation of a private-sector solution to the health care cost problem. The speakers recognized the fact that, to date, the federal program has tended to preempt private initiative. Therefore, renewed commitment of the government to HMO development is coupled with a desire to promote private initiative, not stifle it.

Prescriptions for HEW

The panel in the fourth segment of the conference was devoted to the roles that HEW can assume to advance this objective. Several speakers, representing various interests, presented their ideas on this subject to Under Secretary Hale Champion. Kennett Simmons, Vice President, Health Care Programs, Prudential Insurance Company of America, stressed three roles for HEW. First, the department must articulate public policies and objectives for health care generally. These must be broad enough to stimulate diversity, but narrow enough to allow effective monitoring. Where there are inconsistencies among goals, HEW must set priorities. Second, the department should help create an environment which will encourage private-sector involvement. If activity is to flourish in the private sector, a predictable set of rules and circumstances must be formulated. Third, HEW must act as facilitator and catalyst, not as primary developer.

Bert Seidman, Department of Social Security, AFL-CIO, urged HEW to develop short- and long-range goals for development. He pointed out that because HMOs are essentially community programs, the department should work through the regional offices, which are familiar with local circumstances and area resources. The department should also insure that HMOs are not sabotaged by local health planning agencies. Finally, administration of the department's HMO and related programs should be sufficiently flexible to augment their effectiveness.

James Doherty, Legislative Counsel, Group Health Association of America, suggested that HEW continue to make explicit the federal policy of making a private-sector system work, rather than creating a federal system. As part of this policy, HEW should use its resources both to spur HMO development where there is no local action and to educate the public in an effort to popularize the HMO concept. A major restraint on HMO development is the shortage of qualified personnel, which the department could alleviate through training programs and expanded technical assistance. There is also a danger that the federal program will tend to channel HMOs into the federal models. This should be counteracted by encouraging experimentation with other forms and models of prepaid delivery systems.

The next speaker was Jack Shelton, Manager, Employee Insurance Department, Ford Motor Company. He proposed four areas in which the government can work to eliminate or reduce impediments to HMO development and anticompetitive biases. First, the HMO Act should be revised and regulation reduced to allow HMOs the same flexibility afforded their competitors. For example, the community rating requirement could be eliminated, as well as the requirement for a minimum percentage of practice by physicians in medical groups. Also, the HMO Act could be revised to allow more flexible benefits and to permit greater use of co-payments and deductibles.

Second, HEW should promote greater consistency between programs and agencies. Within its own domain, the department could reduce the burden of certificate-of-need regulations. Also, by trying to persuade the Internal Revenue Service to grant nonprofit HMOs 501 c(3) status, which would make payments to such HMOs tax-deductible, HEW could resolve the tax status issue. The department could also encourage those states which have restrictive HMO laws to make their statutes less onerous.

Third, HEW should promote greater industry and labor involvement in HMOs. Beyond the kinds of educational activities represented by this meeting, the department should work with Congress to alter the incentives in the tax laws so that they encourage purchase of the HMO option.

Finally, HEW should step up its public education activities in an effort to overcome apathy and change public perceptions concerning medical care. Of particular interest would be programs which emphasize the positive aspects of reduced hospitalization and the use of ancillary personnel in delivering high-quality health care.

Robert Biblo, President of the Harvard Community Health Plan, offered several specific recommendations. First, the national health insurance proposals must be carefully monitored to insure that they contain incentives for HMO development; otherwise, such a plan will tend to freeze the system as it presently exists. Second, HEW's policies with respect to all its various programs must be consistent with its policy to work for and support private-sector development of HMOs. Third, a method should be developed to enroll Medicaid and Medicare recipients in HMOs on a capitation, rather than a cost, basis. The resulting savings will accrue to both the government and patients. Fourth, HEW needs to develop criteria for monitoring operational HMOs. As part of this monitoring process, the department should consider reducing regulation of those plans which are successful. And, finally, HEW should use its resources to develop training programs for HMO managers emphasizing practical experience. While there are sufficient numbers of managers having masters degrees in business administration, too few have experience in the HMO setting.

The final speaker on this panel was Dr. Richard Egdahl, Director of Boston University's Center for Industry and Health Care. He suggested that the Office of the Secretary should continue to be involved as a catalyst to maintain the level of commitment. He put forward the idea of developing regional "HMO Development Centers" to offer technical assistance similar to that provided by the regional health planning centers. Beyond serving as an information clearinghouse, each HMO development center could become an effective advocate of the HMO concept, aided by knowledge of the local situation. He also urged HEW to work with the Federal Trade Commission to resolve certain potential problems that face IPAs. In particular, these plans may want to limit the number and mix of specialists in their programs, and many of them use some form of fee schedule. Both practices arouse antitrust concerns which should be dealt with prospectively.

The summary for both this panel and the entire conference was given by Howard Veit, Director, Office of Health Maintenance Organizations, Department of Health, Education, and Welfare. He began by sketching some of the actions HEW plans to take to strengthen the program in response to the kinds of concerns raised by the last panel. He cited the newly centralized HMO office and the expectation that red tape and paperwork will be minimized, thereby reducing the time needed to make decisions. He promised increased monitoring of operational plans as well as a greater effort to enroll Medicaid and Medicare recipients in HMOs on a mutually advantageous basis. Finally, the HMO office will take a more active role in starting HMOs where none now exist.

Veit stressed three points in his summary of the conference. First, business and labor involvement is important to the success of an HMO strategy. Second, HMO support is consistent with business objectives since the heart of any successful HMO is good business practice. Third, HEW must undertake four activities to facilitate the development of HMOs; the department must: (1) devise objectives and strategies and provide resources for HMO development; (2) get business and labor people and money involved in the effort; (3) develop an appropriate training program for HMO managers; and (4) aggressively market the HMO concept to the American people. He expressed his hope that this conference would mark the beginning of a major new effort to create a private-sector solution to the problem of health care costs.

Appendix II

Bay State Health Care Foundation Hearings

Anthony J. Mahler

In early August of 1977, shortly after final HMO regulations had been issued by the Commonwealth's Division of Insurance, the Bay State Health Care Foundation filed an application for a license to operate as an HMO in Massachusetts. The application's single sponsorship surprised the Division, since it had been widely believed that Bay State would file jointly with Blue Shield of Massachusetts, Inc., with which the Foundation had been working since 1974. The filing indicated that Blue Shield would play no role in the proposed HMO.

Instead, the Bay State proposed to use independent contractors to provide the various administrative services it was unable to support on its own: Dikewood Industries for computer and claims processing services, Martin E. Segal Co. for actuarial services, and Frank B. Hall & Co. for marketing services.

The Bay State application raised several important issues and consequently spurred a thorough review by the regulatory agency not only of the Bay State Health Care Foundation, but also of the fee-for-service HMO movement. The ultimate decision rested with the Commissioner of Insurance.

First, the Foundation was proposing the largest fee-for-service HMO in the country, covering all of metropolitan Boston, plus the northeastern corner of Massachusetts and certain areas of the southwest of Boston. The proposed service area included approximately 4,000 practicing physicians and 75 hospitals, ranging from small community facilities to the large teaching hospitals associated with the three Boston medical schools. At the time of its filing, Bay State had some 1,100 participating physicians; in the next few months the figure rose to 1,750. The sheer size and geographical dispersion of the program prompted the Division of Insurance to focus on the control mechanisms proposed by the Bay State.

The Bay State's break with Blue Shield drew attention to a second issue—proposed plans for reimbursing participating physicians. It was assumed by the Division that the break was in part due to the dispute between organized medicine in Massachusetts and Blue Shield over the level of physicians' fees. This dispute had occasioned a class action suit by Massachusetts physicians against Blue Shield, with the outcome still pending. The Division wanted to look at the level of fees proposed by Bay State to determine whether it was consistent with controlling health care costs.

The principal requirement for a license to operate as an HMO in Massachusetts is demonstration of financial viability. Thus, the Bay State marketing and enrollment plan, prepared in conjunction with Frank B. Hall & Co., was a major concern. Unlike most marketing plans for HMOs, which concentrate on large accounts, Hall intended to pursue accounts in the range of 100 to 500 employees. Hall also projected a remarkable success rate for this strategy: enrollments at the end of the first three years of operation were to be 25,000, 75,000, and 125,000, a growth rate unparalleled in HMO history, with penetrations in the enrolled groups approaching 100 percent.

The financial projections were equally optimistic. Positive cash flow was predicted before the end of the first full year of operations. Since both Hall and Dikewood Industries had agreed to be compensated on a per-member basis, virtually all costs would be variable, and the Bay State could operate with a small capital base. Capitalization was derived entirely from a $100-per-physician initiation fee. The assumptions inherent in these financial and marketing plans raised several further issues for the Division staff to explore.

Another important criterion for an HMO license in Massachusetts is sufficient protection of potential HMO members in the presumably unlikely event that the organization folds. Bay State proposed to cover this eventuality through a reinsurance policy with Mutual of Omaha and through contractual agreements with participating physicians and area hospitals. However, given the concerns raised by other portions of the application, Division staff also concentrated on the issue of consumer protection.

Until most of these concerns could be laid to rest the Division hesitated to issue a license to the Bay State Health Care Foundation. After seven months of relatively unproductive negotiations, the two parties agreed to a public hearing on the issues, to be held in May of 1978, with the Commissioner presiding. The Division agreed to issue its final decision on the license as soon after the hearing as possible. The hearing explored in some depth the salient issues raised by the Bay State application: utilization controls, physicians fees, marketing approaches, financial projections, and insolvency protections.

Utilization Controls

The Bay State application proposed the use of retrospective peer review, with appropriate sanctions, as the primary means of insuring that physicians meet projected utilization levels. Bay State also intended to withhold 10 percent of physicians' fees to provide a risk fund. The figure was raised to 20 percent before the hearing. Bay State argued that its experience with Professional Standard Review Organization (PSRO) reviews (the Bay State PSRO is a parallel organization) showed that the Foundation could achieve a satisfactory utilization level with only a retrospective review system like that of the PSRO, although more stringent controls would be adopted if circumstances dictated. In an attempt to diffuse opposition to its proposal, Bay State amended its filing immediately before the hearing to include a preadmission certification program. Bay State also argued that the 20 percent retention of fees would create a reserve fund large enough to cover any excessive utilization.

Division staff argued that Bay State would need to deploy all levels of utilization control from the beginning to be able to control the large number of members projected, Bay State could get into serious financial difficulty before a retrospective review system would flag the trouble, and remedial controls would by that time be too late to be effective. Furthermore, they argued that a 20 percent withholding fund would not give the physicians sufficient incentive to change their practice patterns, and the fund would not cover a large deviation from expected utilization. As witnesses, the Division called Richard Burke, executive director of the Physicians Health Plan of Greater Minneapolis, and Harry Sutton, an actuarial consultant with Stennes Associates. Burke testified primarily about the Minneapolis HMO, which had started with few controls, lost $500,000 in the first year, and been forced to implement drastic controls and increase its holdback to 30 percent in order to bring utilization down to a reasonable level. He did not believe that Bay State could be successful without a concurrent review program and strict sanctions, in addition to the two programs Bay State proposed. Sutton testified that withholding 20 percent of fees would not be sufficient to cover adverse experience; however, he also pointed out that a substantially higher withholding rate would discourage physician participation.

Bay State agreed, during the hearings, to institute the full panoply of utilization control programs as a condition for obtaining a license. However, the Foundation still refused to increase the withholding rate to 30 percent, as requested by the Division, on the grounds that it was unnecessary and would reduce physician participation.

Physicians' Fees

Bay State proposed a reimbursement system for its physicians using a usual, customary, and reasonable approach combined with a maximum fee schedule. Prior to the hearing, Bay State agreed to restrict fee increases to the growth of the consumer price index, exclusive of the medical services component. The Foundation argued that this system would give it sufficient control over the level of fees, while allowing physicians to collect fees that they considered reasonable. In fact, it was suggested in materials sent to the physicians that they could expect to obtain higher fees than they received under Blue Shield, Medicaid, or Medicare; this was used as an inducement for physicians to agree to participate in the Bay State plan.

Opponents argued that this system would tend to inflate, rather than control, physicians' fees. First, they argued that physicians would raise their fees to the maximum level and thus defeat the system. Second, since the maximum fees would be higher than those available under the three major reimbursement programs in Massachusetts, they would contribute to the general inflation of health care costs in the state. Opponents suggested lowering the maximum fee schedule, either by 10 percent, or to the level of Medicare fees plus 5 percent.

Bay State did not agree to follow this recommendation, insisting that its proposed fee schedule was not too high, and that it offered an appropriate incentive for physicians to participate in a program which would, at the same time, restrict their medical practice. Bay State also noted that, in conjunction with the 20 percent withholding rate, the fee schedule would provide lower reimbursement for physicians, unless they were able to meet the utilization targets, since 20 percent of their fees would be forfeited.

Marketing

The marketing strategy prepared by Hall focused on a target group selected according to such factors as existing relationship with Hall, current premium, and size of group. Opponents argued that since Hall's incentive is to maximize enrollment (Hall's reimbursement is a percentage of premium), the company might be tempted to enroll high-risk groups, for whom the Bay State package and premium would be particularly attractive, even though such enrollment would ultimately endanger the plan. The opponents thus recommended that Bay State tighten its controls over the Hall marketing effort. Bay State agreed to adopt written policies governing selection and risk management, to monitor closely the Hall activities, and to retain the right to reject any group proposed by Hall as a marketing target.

Opponents also focused on the unspoken assumptions behind Hall's market penetration estimates and questioned whether Hall and Bay State really intended to market on a dual-choice basis, or rather to offer only the Bay State plan to employees of the enrolled groups. Such a practice would contradict principles of HMO marketing, and might endanger the plan as a result of member dissatisfaction with the lack of choice. Bay State maintained that the plan would be offered on a dual-choice basis, but would be so advantageous as to attract virtually all eligible employees. The Foundation also argued that meeting the enrollment projections was not critical to the financial success of the plan, owing to the high percentage of variable costs.

Financial Structure

The Bay State proposed two major sources of funds to protect the plan against adverse financial performance: initial capitalization of $100 per physician and reserves created by withholding 20 percent of physicians' fees. Bay

State intended to supplement this with a bank line of credit, since its capital had been significantly reduced during the long application period. Arguing that these funds would be insufficient to cover "worst-case" utilization, opponents urged the Commissioner to require that the Bay State raise an additional $800,000 or more, and that it be raised from the individual physicians, with each physician contributing from $750 to $1,500. Beyond providing a solid financial base, such a requirement would insure that the participating physicians were committed to the success of the plan. A $750 minimum contribution would be the largest such fee in any comparable IPA/HMO. (Forty physicians in St. Louis did put up $6,000 apiece to form an IPA, but as an investment in a for-profit organization in which the majority of participating physicians did not contribute funds.)

Bay State replied that it was willing to require an additional $100 from its physicians, but that there was no need to require contributions over $200, since the board of directors could increase the portion of fees withheld in order to cover any "worst-case" experience. Furthermore, such a large contribution requirement would discourage physician participation, and thus impede effective operation of the plan. Opponents agreed that the requirement would discourage physician participation, but contended that a smaller plan, with fewer physicians, would presumably be more manageable and less susceptible to failure.

Insolvency Protection

The reinsurance policy that Bay State purchased from Mutual of Omaha to cover potential insolvency was fairly representative of those available to preoperational HMOs, according to Hall, which investigated the reinsurance market for Bay State. The policy provided that Mutual of Omaha would continue to cover any members hospitalized on the date of insolvency (from the date of insolvency), and would make available to all members a conversion policy without requiring evidence of insurability. In addition, participating physicians would continue to be bound by their contracts to hold patients harmless, and could not bill patients for claims due from Bay State. Bay State agreed to include a similar provision in its contracts with hospitals. Moreover, Bay State assumed that should the plan fail, its members would in most cases be absorbed back into the traditional indemnity insurance plans offered by their employers.

Opponents asserted that members would expect to continue receiving roughly the same level of benefits under a conversion policy, whereas the policy offered by Mutual of Omaha was quite limited. They wanted the Bay State to attempt to obtain a conversion policy with approximately the same level of benefits, or, failing that, to disclose fully to potential members the nature of the conversion policy. Bay State replied that it had been unable to locate such coverage and that the disclosure requirement was discriminatory since a similar requirement had not been made of other licensed HMOs in Massachusetts.

Conclusion

The Commissioner's ruling on the application was delivered on August 31, 1978. In a forty-four page decision, he denied the license for three reasons. First, he found the initial capitalization insufficient, based on the proposed structure, and determined that the contribution per physician should average $1000, rather than the $200 agreed upon during the hearing. Second, he ruled the 20 percent withholding insufficient, and required a 30 percent level. Third, he expressed serious concerns that the Bay State might have an anti-competitive impact on the medical market because of its size and apparent medical society ties. Finally, he said that if Bay State would correct these flaws in its application, and specifically affirm that it would not engage in any anti-competitive practices, a license would be granted without further delay.

The text of the Commissioner's decision addressed certain other issues raised in the hearings, but made no specific findings on them. Uncertainty regarding the effectiveness of Bay State's utilization controls and the admitted problems with the insolvency coverage both strengthened the Commissioner's decision to require a large capitalization and withholding rate. The decision also noted that the Division would closely monitor the level of physicians' fees paid by Bay State if it appeared that an effective marketplace did not exist.

The Board of Directors of the Bay State Health Care Foundation met on September 6, and voted to amend the application to meet the Commissioner's objections. The license was therefore granted on September 14. Bay State began to implement a strategy to sign up participating physicians under the new conditions. Marketing to employers is expected to commence in early 1979.

Appendix III

Panel Discussion: Should Industry Sponsor Fee-for-Service HMOs?

Anthony J. Mahler

As part of the National Conference and Workshop on the IPA-HMO, held in Aspen, Colorado, September 13–15, 1978, four representatives of large industrial corporations discussed their companies' involvement in the development of fee-for-service HMOs. Moderated by Richard H. Egdahl, M.D., director of the Boston University Center for Industry and Health Care, the panel comprised Glen Wegner, M.D., medical director of Boise Cascade, Edward Bernacki, M.D., medical director of United Technologies, John Bauer, supervisor of insurance benefits of Armco Inc., and Charles Ryan, M.D. medical director of the Sun Company. Each panelist briefly presented baseline information summarized in the box and then described the firm's involvement with HMOs generally, and with fee-for-service HMOs specifically, and reasons for its interest in actively promoting fee-for-service HMO development. The remainder of the morning consisted of a lively question and answer period, in which it was possible to cover specific topics in greater detail.

Boise Cascade—Joining Forces with Existing Organizations

Glen Wegner spoke first and said, "concern over spiraling costs has led us to explore the feasibility of a research relationship between the Boise Cascade

BOISE CASCADE CORPORATION
Primary Business:	Wood and Paper Products
Annual Sales:	$2.3 billion
Employees:	35,000
Health Benefit Costs:	$25 million
Monthly Family Premium:	$81
Number of HMO Contracts:	7
Average Monthly Family HMO Premium:	$89

UNITED TECHNOLOGIES CORPORATION
Primary Business:	Jet Aircraft Engines, Elevators and Escalators, Wire and Cable, and Helicopters
Annual Sales:	$5.5 billion
Employees:	138,000 (94,000 Domestic)
Health Benefit Costs:	$55 Million
Monthly Family Premium:	$80–$100 depending on state and group division.
Number of HMO Contracts:	3
Average Monthly Family HMO Premium:	$110 (approx.)

ARMCO INC.
Primary Business:	Steel
Annual Sales:	$3.5 billion
Employees:	51,000 (41,000 Domestic)
Health Benefit Costs:	$60 Million
Monthly Family Premium:	$103
Number of HMO Contracts:	9
Average Monthly Family HMO premium:	$93

SUN COMPANY
Primary Business:	Energy
Annual Sales:	$6.5 billion
Employees:	32,000 (28,000 Domestic)
Health Benefit Cost:	$16.5 million
Monthly Family Premium:	$110
Number of HMO Contracts:	9
Average Monthly Family HMO Premium:	$100, not including the Greater Delaware Valley Health Care, Inc. family premium of $115

Corporation, the Idaho Health Maintenance Organization (a federally-funded IPA-HMO developing in Boise), and the John Hancock Mutual Life Insurance Company, which is the indemnity carrier for Boise Cascade. Our first joint meeting was held in April 1978. We had a long agenda for that meeting, and the issues we faced then are, I believe, the questions that almost any company will have to deal with as they explore such a relationship or try to set up one of these HMOs in their community. They included:

"Why is the Hancock interested in our HMO beyond the fact that Boise Cascade is a major client? And, is Hancock willing to give a 'noncompete' contract to Idaho Health Maintenance Organization so that it wouldn't be taken over by the indemnity carrier at a later date?

"In terms of Boise Cascade's involvement with the HMO, what were the pros and cons of throwing maybe 1,200 people in this community into a model HMO? Would we use the Boise Cascade group for the debugging operation when the HMO opens its doors in 1979?

"In terms of the physician involvement, we talked about medical freedom versus controls, how the doctors are signed up, to what extent are the doctors at risk, how does the patient access the system, what are the limitations of the services, and how is utilization controlled?

"We talked about management information systems, both hardware and software; about financial needs; marketing; insurance coverages such as out-of-area, stop loss, and conversion coverages; actuarial and underwriting services; and where would the Hancock fit into all of these areas.

"We talked about how we could keep GEM Health, a closed panel HMO in Boise, alive; alive but not too prosperous. This really is important, because the biggest impetus we have in our community is the fact that a couple of local family practitioners got together and worked with the federal government to build this GEM Health. This is what got our medical community, which includes some 315 doctors serving 200,000 people, to start the Idaho Health Maintenance Organization.

"Marketing is an issue. Nationally, Boise Cascade has offered seven HMOs with participation ranging from 2 to 13 percent, and an average of 6 percent. Other than the fact that our employees currently have a good group health plan, it is felt that one of the biggest drawbacks to an employee enrolling in an HMO is the cost difference. The Idaho Health Maintenance Organization premium cost will exceed the present cost of providing the Hancock coverage, but only slightly.

"In summary, I think Boise Cascade is taking a major step in the delivery of a health care system to a portion of its employees, but I emphasize that this is a pilot project. We are making an effort to improve the external delivery system. It is our hope that by meeting this issue squarely, we will be able to work more effectively toward bringing the cost of our benifit packages under control."

United Technologies—Considering a Corporate Plan

The next speaker was Edward Bernacki. After summarizing his firm's current health care plan and its costs, he said, "United Technologies is in the process of analyzing whether there are ways we can reduce our expenditures for health care and return some of the savings back to our employees in the form of other types of benefits. We convened a group to look at this question, including the corporate medical director and the director of employee benefits, together with representatives of the treasurer's office and the operations analysis division.

"We began by looking at trends in the costs related to the administration of the benefit and found that they have been stabilized over the past five years at about 6 percent of premium. This suggested to us that we had probably realized most of the savings potential existing in this area and led us to conclude that we would have to focus on the way medical care was being delivered to our employees and their dependents in order to effect a reduction in our medical care costs.

"Since hospital costs accounted for about 60 percent of the total expenditure, we thought it logical to concentrate our efforts on a careful look at employee and dependent hospital utilization. We examined four possible methods to accomplish this—copayments, second surgical opinion, concurrent hospital utilization review, and HMOs—and through a process of elimination arrived at HMOs as the most promising approach for us. Copayment had never been demonstrated to reduce hospitalization, and in any case, would not be a realistic option for us because we have already eliminated copayment from our plan. A second surgical opinion program was added to our plan in April; my preliminary feeling is that we are going to come out behind on it. Concurrent hospital review was instituted in March for Hartford United Technologies employees, but from my reading of the literature I very much doubt that it is going to appreciably reduce our expenditures.

"When we turned to HMOs, we looked at published experiences of both group practice and IPA-HMOs, and were satisfied that their capacity to reduce hospitalization has been pretty well demonstrated. So we engaged a consulting firm to help us assess the benefits and costs of establishing an HMO for our Connecticut population—about 148,000 people counting both employees and their dependents. The analysis took account of the age and sex mix of our population and matched this against populations served by several different types of established HMOs. It was the consultant's judgment that the group practice HMO might achieve about a 55 percent reduction in employee and dependent hospitalization, compared to a 36 percent reduction in an IPA-HMO. When taking account of geography, however, it was predicted that only 10 percent of our population would join a group practice HMO, whereas 50 percent might elect to join an IPA-HMO. This difference in market penetration meant that the overall savings in medical care costs predicted for the two types of HMO were roughly equal. We feel that the IPA has a greater chance of being welcomed or at least accepted by most Connecticut physicians, and the costs involved in starting an IPA are considerably less than start-up costs for the group practice HMO. Moreover, since we already have an extensive in-house medical program involved in preventive health care, a full-scale closed panel HMO would in some ways be duplicative for us. An IPA-HMO built on physicians in the community could take care of curative medicine for our population in a way that would complement our existing services. For example, our in-house laboratories could handle most of the tests ordered by the IPA physicians, and thus achieve significant efficiencies.

"Having taken all of these factors into account, we are now approaching the conclusion that for United Technologies in Connecticut an IPA-HMO may be the most attractive and most feasible mechanism for restraining our health care costs. It still remains for the board to decide whether the corporation will move ahead on this. If we get the green light, we will begin to evaluate the several avenues for implementation that have opened up to us during our preliminary investigations."

Armco, Inc.—A Long-Term Educational Challenge

John Bauer was the third speaker. He sketched the information in the box and added, "Armco, Inc., formerly Armco Steel, has about 40,000 employees across the country, with 20 locations of 500 or more. In the past ten to twelve years our costs for medical care have risen dramatically. As part of doing what we can to control these costs, we are now dealing with approximately twelve HMOs across the country. This involvement dates back only two or three years, and even now only about 2 percent of our people are in HMOs, so we cannot pinpoint exactly what the savings have been or could be. To the extent that HMOs are cheaper, however, the company achieves the savings since Armco fully pays the premiums for a generous standard policy.

"We have wanted to see what we can do to encourage HMOs in locations where we currently have no access to one. In three or four locations across the country we are a dominant employer in the local labor force, and there we feel we may have the leverage to try to encourage physicians to form IPAs. Because these are generally communities of under 50,000 to 60,000 people, though, we don't want to flex our muscles too much in the community and undermine the local medical community. Typically these areas are maybe five to ten years behind the state of the art, which means a very difficult educational process is needed to bring them up to date.

"Two of our locations can serve as examples of what we are doing. One is our corporate headquarters in Middletown, Ohio. About six months ago we began meeting with the doctors to ask them if they would be interested in forming an IPA of their own, and to say that we would encourage or assist them in any way we could. The obvious question that they came back with was, why? There is no outside pressure on them, from a closed panel HMO or anything else. When we look at items such as length of stay or cost per day, Middletown Hospital tends already to be low. This makes it very difficult to persuade the physicians that we need them to begin to do some things.

"The other location is Butler, Pennsylvania just north of Pittsburgh. About a year ago, the new administrator of the local hospital was very interested in forming an IPA-HMO. But when he contacted our local plant and the other two large employers in Butler, he found them unwilling to go out on a limb and commit themselves. More recently—within the past three or four months—I've been in touch with the administrator and we're going to try again. I've contacted some of the other corporate staffs in the area, but the problem is that they have no ability at this point to do anything at a local level. So you can see that we are really at the beginning of this process of trying to find out how to encourage the IPA-HMO in local communities."

Sun Company—Catalyzing a Multiple-Company Effort

Charles Ryan, the final speaker, described a process that has progressed the farthest of the four companies represented. "I am coming at you wearing two hats: that of corporate medical director and that of past chairman of an IPA. At Sun, our reasons for getting involved in developing an IPA are familiar. Rising health care costs and the HMO Act of 1973 prompted a lot of questions from our benefits people. And we were concerned that the federal government might go to national health insurance with the present delivery system, where-upon our cost problems would escalate. So our objective has been to get a system in place now that might enable us to control those costs in the future.

"We are a fairly large corporation, but are capital-intensive and low in numbers of employees. We have only 6,000 employees in Philadelphia, too few for us to go it alone as some of the other panelists have suggested. So we decided to see who else might be interested. Together with twenty other companies we funded a study by a consulting company for an IPA-HMO. The study revealed that three of the six major hospitals in our area and 300 of the 660 physicians were interested in participating and that 87 percent of our employees' families lived within five miles of one of the potential delivery sites. We also found that physicians in our area were in no way interested in a closed panel HMO. We analyzed financial feasibility and found that for 2,000 potential enrollees the premium would be about equal to their current indemnity plans, for 5,000, it would be $10 higher, for 22,000 $10 to $20 higher, and for 35,000, approximately $30 higher. Given the increased services we were planning to offer, we thought we could be competitive.

"We then formed a foundation composed of providers, hospitals, doctors, unions, and industry. But when we came back to the industries for more support, half dropped out. Fortunately ten of them went along and we were able to continue. We set up subcommittees to investigate all the details of what this IPA-HMO would look like. By the time that was over, only our corporation was still willing to contribute more money. So we went to the federal government for a planning grant, and they have given us a lot of help.

"We are now operating, with 300 physicians, and are doing all the things that an IPA has to do to become federally qualified. This we want to do because we plan to offer the IPA to all of the local industries. If we offer it nonqualified, we face two problems. One, the firms now have so many HMOs coming at them that they really don't want to offer an unqualified one. Two, people are worried about what happens if the plan should not make it. As you know, qualified plans are required to cover that contingency. So we definitely want to be qualified."

In summary, the panelists represented a wide range of experience in HMO development. They raised several of the key concerns which occur at nearly any point in a company's HMO development process. How does the company get the physician community "on board," and what should the relationship be? How does an executive get and maintain corporate commitment? What is the role of the current health insurance carrier? And should the company work with other groups or should it plan to "go it alone"?

Discussion

While the discussion period covered a wide range of topics, four areas received particular attention: marketing, unions, disability, and the need for HMO networks. The marketing discussion was started by a question on why a company might choose to push an HMO to its own employees. Wegner answered that, "basically what we want is qualified health care at a reasonable cost, and the assurance that our people will be adequately covered. Working with the Idaho HMO is an opportunity for us to assure that the best doctors in this particular community are taking care of the patients we are interested in."

How Well Can an Employer Market an HMO?

All of the panelists agreed that the attitude of the employer is a key determinant of the penetration achieved by any HMO. For Bernacki, the role of the corporation obviated the need for qualification. He noted that the HMOs with which United Technologies has contracts have penetration rates of about 1–3 percent. "I feel that the poor penetration is due to the fact that the corporation has not been effective in selling an HMO. I am sure that the penetration level would be much higher if we did this." Bauer felt that a first class marketing job by Armco could achieve 20 to 25 percent penetration. Owing to the extensive benefits that his employees already receive, however, he has found that, "the areas that we have seen a large enrollment in HMOs have been those areas where the employees are dissatisfied with the claims procedures of the current carrier. If they are satisfied with the doctors they are going to, and they're getting their claims paid, what's going to get them into an HMO? With our benefit plans there has to be something on the outside getting the employees into the HMO."

Ryan's experience in marketing his IPA suggests that employer attitude is not the whole story: "Our first penetration of our IPA represented three years of work with management and with the unions. Everybody was totally behind us. We had letters encouraging employees to join. We had meetings on company time. We used plan doctors and plan marketing staff as well as management to help us. Our penetration was 5.2 percent of potential enrollees." While there was often a price differential for the employees, the benefits offered were much greater. For one of the companies, the premium was below the HMOs, and penetration was only 2.3 percent. Thus, he feels that price is not the key either: "Our premium right now is $7 more than the current Blue Cross/Blue Shield contract for a family. Even though the union is telling them to take it and management is telling them to take it, people are very reluctant to leave a system that they are comfortable with." United Technologies, however, would plan to offer their HMO with somewhat better benefits at no cost to the employee, and thus feels that a very high penetration rate could be achieved.

What is the Union's Role?

The panel also addressed the question of union involvement in IPAs. Although Wegner has not yet involved his unions in the development process, he sees the IPA as "a middle ground position, not as attractive to the union as national health insurance, but moving in the right direction. We find the unions to be receptive to these ideas." Bauer has also not been in contact with his unions concerning HMOs, but recent Steelworkers' contracts have contained "a statement that if an HMO is available then we as employers are obligated to offer it to the employees. The big problem that we are finding is ignorance about HMOs. The unions have done nothing to educate the employees about what they are."

Ryan involved unions early on in his HMO development effort. "Our original eleven man board had three labor members. After all, our contracts have to be negotiated. Through the education process and working on our board, they understood that they could get better service for at least the same cost, or control costs leaving the money for them to get in wages. So I would not even attempt this without labor and they have been very helpful to us."

Do IPAs Reduce Disability Days?

On the subject of the effects of IPAs on disability days, the panelists were agreed that there is as yet no evidence that there will be a favorable impact, although there was some optimism that this will be the case. Ryan sees this reduction in disability days following from the operation of an IPA: "We lose an awful lot of days in hospitalization and in what we feel is inappropriate care. We think peer review and utilization review may correct this. I am leaving it to the IPA system to do this. The reason we got so involved was to make sure we got a benefits package and the kinds of physicians that we feel can render that kind of care."

Wegner sees some payoff possible owing to the preventive component of an HMO: "The data may be a little soft, but I think there is some suggestion from some of the multiphasic health programs (where there has been periodic reevaluation of employees) that there has been some reduced absenteeism and maybe some increased productivity. The worried well become reassured, don't go to doctors as often, and don't sit around on the job worrying about what might be wrong with them. I don't think the data is complete but its worth following." Bauer also raised the point that simply getting the employee into a more organized system of care might reduce disability and absenteeism. Bernacki proposes that the IPA could be designed to reduce disability days: "Perhaps there could be some sort of incentive system set up to encourage physicians to return employees back to work as soon as their medical conditions permit."

Disincentives to Involvement—Management Headaches

Finally, the panel posed the special problem faced by large corporations in dealing with HMOs. Wegner outlined his situation: "We have a management information system for employees that is very efficient and is used across the country. But when we go on these HMO contracts we have to deal with the data manually. And the other thing is that we have a lot of transfers since our employees are upwardly mobile within the company. Currently we can handle the insurance transfer in 30 seconds for someone under our Hancock coverage by calling it up on the scope. But we can't do that for the HMOs. If we don't have some uniformity in coverages and transferability, its going to be yet another serious barrier to increased competitive enrollment. I see the need for some national organization to serve a linking role. We are going to need standardized benefits, the benefits our employees want and the ones which the unions have negotiated. Our function will be to subcontract with the best HMOs who will provide our package so we can get back to our single employee information system."

In summary, this panel presented the experiences of four large corporations as they have become actively involved in fee-for-service HMO development, and highlighted some of the challenges that they are facing. Wegner from Boise Cascade discussed an innovative approach to working with an insurance carrier to encourage HMO development. Bauer from Armco explored the difficulty of working in smaller communities where there is no credible threat from a group practice HMO. Bernacki from United Technologies laid out a plan to establish an in-house fee-for-service HMO designed to build on the company's extensive medical resources. And Ryan from Sun was able to provide a "real world" perspective as one who has played a central role in the development of a fee-for-service HMO.